Advances in
Health Education

ABOUT THE EDITORS

Robert H. L. Feldman is Professor and Director of the Program in Health Behavior, Department of Health Education, University of Maryland, College Park. Previously, he was on the faculty of Johns Hopkins University, School of Hygiene and Public health. Dr. Feldman has published extensively in the areas of health behavior, health psychology, and worksite health (including co-editor of Advances in Health Education: Current Research, Volumes 2 and 3, and co-authorship of Occupational Health Promotion: Health Behavior in the Workplace)

James H. Humphrey, Professor Emeritus at the University of Maryland, is the author of more than 46 books and 200 articles and research reports. Ten of his books have been concerned with the areas of health and health education. A notable researcher, he was a charter member and first chairman-elect of the Research Council of the American School Health Association.

ADVANCES IN HEALTH EDUCATION

Current Research
Volume 4

Edited by
Robert H. L. Feldman
and
James H. Humphrey

AMS PRESS, INC.
New York

ADVANCES IN HEALTH EDUCATION: *Current Research*

Copyright ©1996 by AMS Press, Inc.

ISSN 0890-4073

Series ISBN: 0-404-63550-4
Vol. 4 ISBN: 0-404-63554-7

Library of Congress Catalog Card Number: 86-47857

All AMS books are printed on acid-free paper that meets the guidelines for performance and durability of the Committee on Production Guidelines for Book Longevity of the Council on Library Resources.

AMS Press, Inc.
56 East 13th Street
New York, N.Y. 10003

Manufactured in the United States of America

CONTENTS

PREFACE

The fourth volume of *Advances in Health Education* presents a selection of current research and state-of-the-art research reviews. The field of health education continues to exhibit multidisciplinary trends and the present volume reflects this diversity.

This volume examines such topics as HIV/AIDS prevention programs and adolescent sexuality. The increasing interest of health educators in these issues is reflected in this volume. Preventive health behaviors are investigated among different age groups in the United States and among rural workers in Argentina. Exercise and physical activity is addressed in studies of college students and older adults. In addition, the fourth volume contains selections on high school health education, worksite smoking cessation programs, and methodological issues in health education.

In conjunction with AMS Press we intend to provide health education students and researchers with an annual series reporting original research investigating factors concerned with human health and health education. The volumes are intended to supplement and support journals reporting on similar topics. Papers eligible for inclusion in this and subsequent volumes must be (a) previously unpublished original research studies investigating selected aspects of health education, (b) state-of-the-art research reviews on topics of current interest with a substantial research literature base, or (c) theoretical papers presenting well-formulated but as yet untested models.

A volume of this nature would not be possible without the cooperation of many individuals. In this regard we wish to thank the contributors for presenting their work. In addition, we express our gratitude to the distinguished board of reviewers for giving their valuable time and excellent talents to this endeavor.

CONTRIBUTORS

C. Alexander, Johns Hopkins University School of Hygiene & Public Health, Baltimore, Maryland

Dean Anderson, Iowa State University, Ames, Iowa

Mary Lou Balassone, University of Washington, Seattle, Washington

J. Baldwin, Johns Hopkins University School of Hygiene & Public Health, Baltimore, Maryland

Michelle A. Bell, University of Washington, Seattle, Washington

Lillian Cook Carter, Towson State University, Towson, Maryland

Vivien C. Carver, University of Southern Mississippi, Hattiesburg, Mississippi

Charles M. Cychosz, Iowa State University, Ames, Iowa

Michael R. Davey, Western Illinois University, Macomb, Illinois

Thomas E. Deeter, Iowa State University, Ames, Iowa

Ruth C. Engs, Indiana University, Bloomington, Indiana

Richard I. Evans, University of Houston, Houston, Texas

Robert H.L. Feldman, University of Maryland, College Park, Maryland

M. Fowler, Johns Hopkins University School of Hygiene & Public Health, Baltimore, Maryland

Gaston Godin, School of Nursing, Laval University, Sainte-Foy (Quebec), Canada

Walter Greene, Temple University, Philadelphia, Pennsylvania

Roberta B. Hollander, Howard University, Washington, D.C.

Josefa Ippolito-Shepherd, National Institutes of Health, Bethesda, Maryland

Catherine A. Kennedy, Exercise and Sports Science, Colorado State · University

Mark J. Kittleson, Southern Illinois University, Carbondale, Illinois

Ella P. Lacey, Suthern Illinois University, Carbondale, Illinois

Jean Lambert, Department of Social and Preventive Medicine, Universite de Montreal, Montreal (Quebec), Canada

Phyllis M. Levenson-Gingiss, University of Houston, Houston, Texas

M.C. Joelle Fignole Lofton, University of Maryland, College Park, Maryland

Joanne Otis, Department of Social and Preventive Medicine, Universite de Montreal, Montreal (Quebec), Canada

J. Pankey, Central Maryland Chapter of the American Red Cross, Baltimore, Maryland

M. Perry, Johns Hopkins University School of Hygiene & Public Health, Baltimore, Maryland

Nancy Peterfreund, Seattle-King County Department of Public Health, Seattle, Washington

M. Platt, Johns Hopkins University School of Hygiene & Public Health, Baltimore, Maryland

Murray A. Preston, University of Houston, Houston, Texas

J. Rolf, Johns Hopkins University School of Hygiene & Public Health, Baltimore, Maryland

Sandra M. Schleiffers, Department of Computer Science, Colorado State University, Ft. Collins, Colorado

Rickard A. Sebby, Southeast Missouri State University, Cape Girardeau, Missouri

William E. Snell, Southeast Missouri State University, Cape Girardeau, Missouri

John S. Venglarcik, Hospital Epidemiologist, Western Reserve Care System, Youngstown, Ohio

David C. Wiley, Southwest Texas State University, San Marcos, Texas

Roberta Hollander, Ph.D.
Associate Professor of Health
  Education
Department of Health,
  Physical Education and
  Recreation
Howard University
Washington, D.C.

Cheryl L. Perry, Ph.D.
Associate Professor
Division of Epidemiology
University of Minnesota
Minneapolis, Minnesota

Renee Royak-Schaler, Ph.D.
Assistant Professor
Department of Health Sciences
Towson State University
Towson, Maryland

John R. Seffrin, Ph.D.
Chairman and Professor
Department of Health and
  Safety Education
Indiana University
Bloomington, Indiana

1

HIV/AIDS PREVENTION PROGRAMS FOR ADOLESCENTS: ENHANCING AND EVALUATING AN EFFECTIVE SCHOOL-BASED EXAMPLE

J. Baldwin
J. Rolf
C. Alexander
M. Platt
M. Perry
M. Fowler
J. Pankey

This chapter describes the background, the processes involved in the development and implementation, and the results of a large scale evaluation study of one of the most widely used HIV/AIDS education curricula - The American Red Cross HIV/AIDS Prevention Program for Youth. In the first part of the chapter, we review the evidence that explains why adolescents are potentially at risk for HIV/AIDS, including findings from relevant descriptive and intervention studies. In the second part, we describe how we chose promising theory-based interventions and assessments in order to enhance and evaluate the Red Cross program and foster preventive behavior changes among youth in our sample of ninth graders. Next, we present our collaborative approach to the implementation of the school-based interventions and evaluations. An overview of findings concerning intervention effects are reported with particular attention to changes in attitudinal and behavioral variables. These outcomes include reports of sex-related HIV-risking behaviors, HIV/AIDS knowledge, self-efficacy beliefs, and preventive communications about HIV/AIDS. We conclude with discussions of the adaptability of the Red Cross HIV/AIDS Prevention Program and our experimental enhancements to local school contexts and different subgroups of students.

AIDS (Acquired Immune Deficiency Syndrome) is now beginning to pose an immense threat to the health of the general public. As of February 28, 1990, the cumulative number of reported AIDS cases in the U.S. was 124,984 (Centers for Disease Control, 1990). More alarmingly, it is estimated that there are 1.0 to 1.5 million people in the U.S. who are **currently** infected with Human Immunodeficiency Virus (HIV-1), the causal agent of AIDS. The Centers for Disease Control (CDC) continues to predict increases in new silent infections as well as AIDS cases. Within two years, the number of AIDS cases is expected to total more than 270,000 and the number of AIDS-related deaths more than 179,000 (Tolsman, 1988).

Concern for the AIDS epidemic threatening the **general population** is a new phenomenon. The early U.S. projections were based on rates of deaths and new infections occurring among the subpopulations originally at highest risk for HIV infection in the United States - homosexual men and intravenous drug users (IVDUs). Even up to the mid- to late 1980s, many epidemiologists and policy makers failed to recognize alternative behavioral bridges that could spread HIV as a sexually transmitted disease among the general U.S. public. Fear, prejudice, religious proscriptions and pressure from lobbies for existing biomedical research funding priorities slowed the nation's receptivity to mounting a meaningful national plan for HIV/AIDS prevention (Watkins, 1988). As a consequence, the first national HIV/AIDS education campaigns in the U.S. were intentionally made much less explicit and more tentative than those in other countries (Liskin, Church, Piotrow & Harris, 1989). During the 1980s, however, there arose a growing number of health educators and researchers who began to explore how cognitive, affective and behavioral attributes of different demographic groups might influence vulnerabilities to HIV/AIDS and receptivity to preventive interventions. Early U.S. survey studies have demonstrated that although most U.S. citizens have learned many of the basic facts about HIV/AIDS, there has been little evidence that increases in AIDS knowledge have led to the practice of preventive behaviors among heterosexuals.

This chapter focuses on adolescents, a subpopulation which may potentially represent one of the next "hot spots" in the AIDS epidemic, largely due to developmentally and culturally normative high rates of unprotected intercourse and experimentation with drugs (Brooks-Gunn, Boyer, Hein, 1988; Rolf, Nanda, Baldwin, Chandra & Thompson, 1990; Washington Post, 1989). Adolescent AIDS cases have only recently been distinguished from adult cases in the reported statistics. As of February, 1990, reported AIDS cases among adolescents represented only 1% of all cases, or 486 adolescents aged 13 to 19 years (CDC, 1990). Similarly, the estimates for adolescents' HIV seroprevalence rates in the U.S. general population are fairly low - one per 1000 among military recruits and two per 1000 among college students (Sonenstein, Pleck, & Ku, 1989). However, it is well known that 21% of all AIDS cases have been diagnosed in the 20-29 age group. Given the long incubation period between HIV infection and the appearance of symptoms leading to the diagnosis of AIDS (an average of 5-7 years), many people developing AIDS in their 20s were likely exposed to the virus when they were teenagers (Hein, 1989).

In an attempt to estimate the potential spread of HIV infection among adolescents, Brooks-Gunn et al. (1988) have suggested the following indicators: (1) the percentage of teenagers who have intercourse only once, (2) the frequency with which youth have intercourse, (3) the number of sexual partners they have, and (4) whether teens have been in contact with persons engaging in HIV-risking behaviors. The rationale for looking at these indicators is apparent: as HIV becomes more prevalent in the general population, risk for exposure from sexual transmission becomes a function of the age of sexual initiation, the number and types of partners, contraceptive and prophylactic practices, and experimentation with drugs. The existing literature on adolescents consists of important sources of information on these HIV/AIDS relevant variables.

Initiation of Sexual Intercourse

Many adolescents have had sexual intercourse by age 16 or 17. However, for some subgroups of teens, the average age of first intercourse has been reported to be as low as 12 years of age (Clark, Zabin, & Hardy, 1984). Also, many adolescents engage in sexual activity quite frequently; among teens 15 years of age and older, 33% or more report having sex at least once a week (Hofferth & Hayes, 1987).

Number of Partners

A substantial proportion of sexually active youth may have had multiple sexual partners. In Sorenson's survey of American adolescents conducted in the 1970s, about 41% of sexually experienced adolescent males reported having more than three partners in the past month, and 13% of sexually experienced adolescent females reported having a total of 17 partners by age 19 (Sorenson, 1973; cited in Hein, 1989). In the 1980s, over 50% of sexually active adolescents reported already having two or more partners (Zelnik, 1983). As noted by some researchers, adolescents who initiate sexual intercourse at younger ages (less than or equal to 14 years) may be more likely to have a greater number of partners during their reproductive years than those adolescents who delay sexual activity (DiClemente, 1989). In addition, adolescents who become sexually involved with *older* individuals (who may have had numerous sexual partners) may be at increased risk of exposure to HIV. Indeed, on average, female adolescents tend to have sexual partners who are 2 to 3 years older than they are (Vermund, Hein, Gayle, Cary, Thomas & Drucker, 1989).

Contraceptive and Prophylactic Practices

Knowledge of the rates of contraceptive practices among sexually active youth is also necessary to assess adolescents' risk for acquisition of HIV/AIDS. According to Zelnik and Shah (1983), approximately 50% of all teenagers do not use contraceptives the first time they have sexual intercourse, with younger adolescents much less likely to use contraceptives than older ones. Of those who use a birth control method, male methods (condoms and withdrawal) appear to be the preferred methods, for both males and females, Blacks and Whites (Brooks-

Gunn et al., 1988). Unfortunately, "the fact that perhaps as many as one half of all teens do not use contraception the first time they have intercourse is not a one-time event" (Brooks-Gunn et al., 1988, p. 960). Young adolescents are more likely than older teens to delay using birth control methods for up to a year after their first sexual experience (Brooks-Gunn & Furstenberg, 1989). These delays may prove to have important consequences, as half of all first pregnancies occur in the first six months following sexual initiation (Zabin, Kantner, & Zelnik, 1979; cited in Brooks-Gunn & Furstenberg, 1989).

Drug Use

The transmission of the AIDS virus has been clearly tied to drug use where needle-sharing serves as the vector of viral spread. Drug use may also be linked to increased probability of sexual transmission of HIV via social association with the drug culture (Shafer, 1988), and/or risky practices during recreational drug use. For example, a study of 248 incarcerated juveniles showed significant associations between HIV-risking behaviors and (1) types and quantities of drug used, (2) getting drunk or high before sex, and (3) availability of alcohol and/or drugs at social gatherings (Rolf et al., 1990). Although illicit drug use seems to be declining slowly among high school seniors, about 1% still report having used heroin and 13% report having used cocaine (Johnston, Bachman, & O'Malley, 1987). As noted by Brooks-Gunn et al. (1988), however, these data probably underestimate the use of drugs by U.S. teens in the general population, principally because in areas of high HIV prevalence, such as urban neighborhoods, the high school dropout rate may be quite high; and higher rates of drug use and of sexual contact with drug users are more prevalent among dropouts than high school seniors.

HIV/AIDS DESCRIPTIVE AND PREVENTIVE INTERVENTION RESEARCH RELEVANT TO ADOLESCENTS

There are a growing number of reports of evaluated HIV/AIDS prevention programs targeting youth. Most of the programs conducted in schools have assessed changes in HIV/AIDS knowledge. Few studies have attempted to measure behavioral change and intention to change. Findings from both HIV/AIDS descriptive and preventive intervention studies will be briefly reviewed here.

Survey Studies of Adolescents' HIV/AIDS Knowledge

A number of descriptive surveys of adolescents' knowledge, attitudes and beliefs about AIDS have been undertaken (e.g., DiClemente, Boyer, & Morales, 1988; DiClemente, Zorn, & Temoshok, 1986; Kegeles, Adler, & Irwin, 1988; Price, Desmond, & Kukulka, 1985; Reuben, Hein & Drucker, 1988; Strunin & Hingson, 1987). These studies demonstrate that even though most teenagers know the basic facts about HIV/AIDS, many youth still hold misconceptions about HIV transmission and engage in behaviors that potentially put them at risk for HIV infection. One of the earliest published reports of 250 junior high and high school students in Ohio indicated that most students had some information about AIDS, but the best informed students answered only 47% of the questions correctly (Price et al., 1985). A large scale study of White, Black, and Latino high school students in the San Francisco Bay area also found that although most adolescents knew that sexual intercourse and sharing needles were major HIV transmission routes (92.4% and 81.1% of the sample knew these facts, respectively), more than a third of the 1326 students incorrectly believed that AIDS could be contracted by shaking hands with or being near someone with AIDS (DiClemente et al., 1986). More alarming was the finding that only 60% of this sample was aware that using condoms during sexual intercourse reduced the risk of disease transmission. Black and Hispanic youth in this sample knew less about AIDS and had more misconceptions about HIV transmission than White students (DiClemente et al., 1988). There is emerging evidence that other minority groups (e.g., Native American youth - Rolf, Alexander, Chandra & Baldwin, 1989; Estrada, Dalgarn, M. de Boer, Fernandez, Stone & Englander, 1989) may also be less knowledgeable about HIV/AIDS and misperceive their personal risks and responsibilities for adopting protective behaviors. Fortunately, a consistent finding across many of these surveys has been that adolescents have reported wanting to learn more about AIDS, particularly, in the school setting.

A number of survey researchers have suggested that youth seem to have distorted perspectives of their own vulnerability to HIV/AIDS. Melton (1988) has discussed the relatively poor risk perception skills of adolescents perhaps attributable to the long latency period between HIV infection and the onset of visible AIDS symptoms. In a study conducted in New York City, the youth engaging in the highest risk sexual behavior perceived themselves to be at lowest risk and did not use protective measures during sexual intercourse (Reuben et al., 1988; cited in Brooks-Gunn et al., 1988). Similarly, Price et al. (1985) found that individuals who were most sexually active were less likely to perceive themselves at risk of infection. Research addressing HIV/AIDS risk perceptions among adolescents is complex. Perloff's (1987) model involving variables of social distance and risk perception is beginning to be applied (Baldwin, Rolf, Pankey, Alexander, Fowler, Perry, & Platt, 1989). Preliminary findings suggest that personal risk is highly correlated with the risks attributed to one's closest friends and family members.

For a majority of adolescents, there is little evidence that knowledge about HIV/AIDS is, in itself, sufficient to promote behavior change. Available data suggest that although some adolescents have reported changes in casual behavior because of fear of AIDS, few have reported changes in sexual activities that actually transmit the virus. For example, a random sample of 860 Massachusetts youth aged 16-19 revealed that while 70% reported they were sexually active, only 15% of them reported changing their sexual behavior because of concern about exposure to

HIV/AIDS, and only 20% of those who changed their behavior used effective methods (Strunin & Hingson, 1986). Kegeles et al. (1988) also found that although most teenagers in a San Francisco study knew that condoms could prevent sexually transmitted diseases, only 2% of sexually active teenage girls and 8% of boys used condoms *every* time they had intercourse. Further, the study revealed that many of the teens had more than one sex partner over a one-year period, and that 10-20% of the sexually active teens had engaged in unprotected anal intercourse (considered one of the highest HIV-risking sexual behaviors).

In a more recent study conducted by Goodman and Cohall (1989), more teenagers (39% vs. 15% in Strunin & Hingson's study) claimed behavior change, and a much larger proportion (82% compared to 20% in Strunin & Hingson, 1986) reported using condoms or practicing abstinence. In addition, those adolescents who claimed to have made a behavior change tended to perceive themselves at greater risk, worry more about the disease, and be more knowledgeable about HIV/AIDS. Of those claiming current condom use, however, only 64% reported using condoms at last sexual intercourse. Females accounted for only 35% of those who claimed such a change. The present authors agree with Goodman and Cohall (1989) that females in this sample demonstrated a lack of *insistence* on condom use despite their high knowledge about means of risk reduction. Therefore, it would appear that HIV/AIDS prevention programs with outcome objectives focused on behavior change must consist of mechanisms to convert knowledge-informed intentions into practice of health behaviors.

HIV/AIDS Preventive Intervention Studies with Adolescents

In response to the threat HIV/AIDS poses to youth in this country, at least 28 states have passed legislation or school certification requirements which mandate HIV/AIDS education in their schools (Kenney, Guardado, & Brown, 1989). In addition, all but four states and virtually every large school district have attempted to adopt some form of AIDS education. However, because AIDS educational materials are still relatively new or still being field tested, little specific information is available on the content, process and especially the effectiveness of these prevention curricula. Furthermore, as mentioned, most evaluations of AIDS education programs to date have focused only on detecting changes in *knowledge* and *attitudes,* while very little longitudinal information has been gathered on the effectiveness of school-based AIDS educational programs in reducing HIV-risking behaviors and promoting protective ones.

Program Impact on HIV/AIDS Knowledge

Significant increases in knowledge *have* been observed when measured before and immediately after AIDS educational programs. For example, in a study by DiClemente, Pies, Stoller, et al. (1989), there was a substantial increase in knowledge among students in the AIDS instruction group about the efficacy of using condoms to prevent HIV infection. At baseline, about 70% of the adolescents correctly reported that condoms could reduce their risk of HIV infection. At posttest, after three consecutive days of AIDS education, almost 92% of the instruction group was aware of the protective value of condoms.

In another relatively early report (Miller & Downer, 1987; cited in U.S. Congress, 1988). AIDS knowledge increased considerably, and students' perceptions regarding personal risk of HIV infection decreased slightly following an AIDS curriculum. Brown, Fritz and Barone (1989) also reported that following an AIDS educational program, 7th- and 10th-grade students demonstrated more knowledge about HIV/AIDS, greater tolerance of AIDS patients, and more hesitancy toward high-risk behaviors, although these changes were considered modest. There is other evidence, as well, which suggests that youth who have *not* participated in HIV/AIDS educational interventions overestimate both the number of AIDS cases and the probability of getting HIV/AIDS from a "single unprotected act of heterosexual intercourse" (Freimuth, Edgar, & Hammond, 1987; cited in U.S. Congress, 1988). Until more data from AIDS education evaluations are available, it is worthwhile to examine the effectiveness of intervention programs that have attempted to reduce teenage pregnancy, educate youth about sex, and reduce smoking and experimentation with alcohol and drugs among teens.

EFFECTIVENESS OF OTHER RELATED HEALTH PROMOTION PROGRAMS FOR ADOLESCENTS

Teen Pregnancy and Sexuality Education

Eighty percent of the states in the United States either require or encourage the teaching of sex education in the public schools, and nearly 90% of large school districts across the U.S. support such instruction (Kenney et al., 1989). However, the prerogatives of community school boards, the amount of time devoted to the programs, and the comprehensiveness and intensiveness of the programs differ widely (Brooks-Gunn et al., 1988). In addition, most school districts place greater emphasis on disease prevention than on pregnancy prevention (Kenney et al., 1989). Particularly relevant for the practice of preventive behaviors, few school districts include decision-making about sexuality as an objective of the program, and the majority of programs are short (10 hours or less) (Kirby, 1984).

In general, sex education has increased factual knowledge about sexuality and sexually transmitted diseases among teens, but has led to little change in attitudes and behavior (Kirby, 1984; cited in U.S. Congress, 1988). Specifically, data from the National Survey on Family Growth suggest that effects of these education programs are not related to changes in sexual behavior, such as reduced frequency of "unsafe" sexual intercourse or lower adolescent pregnancy rates (Hayes, 1987). This might be partly attributed to the fact that few studies have adequately addressed communication and other social skills considered important mediators of sex-related behavior change. Indeed, Flora and Thoresen (1988) assert that a focused skills-training approach has been absent in almost all classroom or school-based efforts. As these authors explain, students are not usually taught the behavioral and cognitive skills one must possess to know how to use contraceptives or how to resist pressure to have sex.

One exceptional study which included training in relevant cognitive and behavioral skills was that conducted by Gilchrist and Schinke (e.g., Gilchrist & Schinke, 1983; Schinke, 1984). One of their interventions consisted of 14 sessions of intensive cognitive-behavioral training employing role playing and rehearsal to enhance communication skills and attitudes crucial to lowering risk of pregnancy. Six months after the intervention, the participants reported using more effective contraceptive methods and demonstrated better communication skills than members of the control group.

Other Preventive Intervention Programs Targeting Adolescents

The work conducted with young adolescents in the fields of smoking and substance abuse prevention have been particularly informative (e.g., Botvin, 1986; Flay, 1987; Flora & Thoresen, 1988; Glynn, Leukfeld & Ludford, 1983; Killen, McAlister, Perry, & Maccoby, 1982; NIDA, 1986). These behavioral and peer group-oriented programs have demonstrated some promising decreases in initiation of smoking and substance use. We concur with the conclusions of a report from the Office of Technology Assessment of the U.S. Congress (1988) that programs most likely to succeed in changing adolescents' health related behavior are those that "relate information to their personal situations and that use techniques such as role playing to teach *communication skills* and to reinforce new *peer group norms*" (p. 8).

THE HARFORD COUNTY MARYLAND-
RED CROSS HIV/AIDS PREVENTION PROGRAM
FOR YOUTH EVALUATION PROJECT

The present project was specifically designed to build on the theoretical and practical aspects of previous research with adolescents that has identified how normative attitudes and behaviors are involved in impeding or facilitating health behavior changes. The purpose of the project was to test the effectiveness of the widely used American Red Cross HIV/AIDS Prevention

Program for Youth and as well as three additional experimental interventions which were hypothesized to enhance the impact of the Red Cross program on students' preventive intentions and behaviors. This project was conducted as a collaborative effort involving the Central Maryland Chapter of the American Red Cross, the Harford County Maryland Public School System and the Johns Hopkins School of Hygiene and Public Health. The project's specific outcome and process objectives are listed in Table 1.

Aspects of the Health Belief Model (HBM) (Janz & Becker, 1984) and Social Learning Theory (SLT) (Bandura, 1986a, 1986b) that have produced useful information in previous research were incorporated into two of the experimental interventions and the attendant pre, post and follow-up assessments. (In the Methods Section, Table 3 lists the categories of variables measured in our project.) From the HBM, *perceived barriers* (e.g., embarrassment, peer-norms of health-risking and non-preventive behaviors) were more intensively assessed than *perceived susceptibility* to HIV/AIDS and *perceived benefits* of preventive behaviors (e.g., benefits of using condoms). Previous SLT based interventions (e.g., the work by Gilchrist, Schinke and colleagues) have pointed to the importance of *self-efficacy* beliefs as key variables in coping with perceived barriers and skill-building practice prior to achieving the expected beneficial outcomes. Therefore, we "enhanced" the Red Cross program with experimental intervention components involving peer modeling and reinforced practice of communication about (1) assessing HIV-STD and pregnancy risks in social encounters, (2) resisting pressures for unwanted and unsafe behaviors; and (3) asserting health promoting alternatives. These interventions, the research design and assessment strategies used to evaluate their effects, and the discussion of key findings are presented next.

METHODS

Evaluation Design

As seen in Figure 1, the project used a quasi-experimental design to compare intervention effects for two student cohorts within schools, as well as *between* similar pairs of schools. Schools 1 & 3, and Schools 2 & 4 were matched on basic sociodemographic characteristics. Semester cohorts provided opportunities for within and between school replications as one-half of the ninth graders were assigned by school scheduling personnel to a Fall-health education/Spring-physical education sequence, while the other half was assigned to a reverse sequence (Fall-physical education and Spring-health education). As explained in more detail later, the *core* HIV/AIDS educative intervention evaluated both semesters was the American Red Cross HIV/AIDS Prevention Program for Youth. The Harford County Teen Pregnancy Unit is usually taught just before the Red Cross HIV/AIDS Prevention Program for Youth (abbreviated RC). However, because we hypothesized that the Teen Pregnancy unit (TP) might be "priming" students for the Red Cross HIV/AIDS Prevention Program (and therefore serving as an enhancer), the sequence of the two units was switched during the Spring semester. This switching (i.e., Fall=TP-RC to Spring=RC-TP) enabled us to test for an order effect. Thus, all 4 schools both semesters received the RC and the TP Units, but in a different sequence.

Two additional experimental interventions (1) peer modeling video and role play activity and (2) a photonovel were introduced in the Spring semester. The two enhanced intervention schools conducted the HIV risk-reducing role playing activities as part of the last two sessions of the AIDS Unit. The photonovel was developed and distributed after the AIDS Unit in School 1 only. A fifth school requested permission to join the study during 2nd semester. We were pleased with this further indication of acceptance by the school system and developed two special research purposes for involving this school. The first was to conduct a comparison of the two American Red Cross HIV/AIDS videos "A Letter from Brian" vs. "Don't Forget Sherrie." The second reason was to have this school serve as a second semester comparison for the effects of multiple testing. Schools 1, 2, 3, and 4 (2nd semester) had baseline and three subsequent assessments, while School 5 had *no* baseline but did have the latter three assessments coinciding with the immediate posttest, and the two and eight month follow-ups.

Study Population and Sample

Locale. As indicated, the study took place in Harford County, MD which is located north of the Baltimore, Maryland suburbs and extends northward to the Pennsylvania border. Harford County has been previously considered a rural area but is now rapidly developing into suburban and town-based communities. It has experienced nearly a 26% increase in population over the past 10 years. The total population of Harford County in 1989 was 163,300 of which approximately 9.7% were ethnic minorities. As of November 30th, 1989, 29 AIDS cases had been reported in Harford County. Nine of these 29 cases were among young adults, 20-29 years of age. Harford County ranks sixth highest for reported AIDS cases among Maryland's 24 counties including Baltimore City (AIDS Administration, 1990). Harford County high school principals have cited two AIDS deaths among their recent graduates.

School Participation. Support from the principals, teachers, and parents was essential to the success of the project. To gain the school system's support, preliminary informational discussions were held among representatives from Harford County schools superintendent's staff, the Central Maryland Chapter of the American Red Cross, and the Hopkins research team. After establishing our mutual interest in pursuing a collaborative evaluation project, the prototype surveys developed by the research team, as well as the process for implementation of the project, were reviewed and approved by the Supervisor of Curriculum and the Supervisor of Health and High School Physical Education. Meetings were then held with all of the principals and health education teachers to explain the project's purpose and to gain their support. Annotated versions (i.e., explaining the reasons why each type of question was being asked) of the Fall and Spring semester surveys were also prepared for review by interested parents. Principals mailed an informational letter and consent forms to parents and invited them to review the surveys, and/or to attend parent meetings with both school personnel and research team members present to answer questions. Additional contact for informed consent was made with parents of the students who participated in the development of the photonovel and role play demonstration video.

Student Participation. In total, 1173 health education students participated in the study during the 1988-89 academic year from five of the eight high schools in Harford County Maryland. These five schools were recruited based on their representativeness of the County's student body and their principals' and health education teachers' interest in participating in the study. Students were eligible to participate if they (1) were currently enrolled in health education class, (2) had obtained written consent from their parent(s) and, (3) provided their own written consent on a separate form. As seen in Figure 2, 979 9th-graders (the primary target group) participated in the study. Four hundred and five 9th-graders were surveyed from 4 schools first semester, while 573 9th-graders were surveyed from 5 schools and 2nd semester. Both first and second semesters, students of one school (School 1 then School 5) received posttests only to control for testing effects.

Table 2 illustrates sociodemographic data for the 1st and 2nd Semester cohorts of 9th-graders in our sample by school. On average, half of the subjects were male, most were about 14 years of age, and the majority were White youth of working to middle class families who were attending a centralized high school associated with a rural or suburban township.

Student Participation Over Time. Approximately 92% of all eligible 9th-grade students in the health education courses provided the dual written informed consent and were present to complete the baseline questionnaire. Of these, 84.8% of 1st semester students (262/309) and 88.8% of 2nd semester students (389/438) were present for all three occasions the questionnaires were administered each semester. In addition, six- and eight-month follow-ups were obtained for 85.5% of 1st and 78.8% of 2nd semester 9th-grade cohorts, respectively. Differences in attrition rates for follow-up can be largely attributed to school transfers which occurred during the summer interval. Students of the 2nd semester cohort were surveyed in the Fall of their 10th grade year. At the same time, one year follow-ups were obtained for the 1st semester cohort with 77.6% successfully surveyed.

Program Description: The Interventions

The Core Curriculum. In 1987, the Harford County Board of Education adopted the *Red Cross HIV/AIDS Prevention Program for Youth* for use in ninth grade health education classes. This curriculum package includes a 29-minute video entitled "A Letter From Brian," a workbook, and a teachers/leaders guide; it also has a parent brochure which was not used in the present study. Since its inception, the RC HIV/AIDS program was taught by the Harford County School's health education teachers in five consecutive class periods during the county's semester long ninth grade health education curriculum. Overall, the county teachers have reported being very pleased with the materials. However, in 1988 they recommended developing more classroom activities that might stimulate student discussion. The experimental interventions of the present project were designed to meet this request.

Enhancement 1

Teen Pregnancy Curriculum Unit. Since 1972, the Harford County Public School System has been teaching a Family Life and Human Development program which spans elementary, middle, and high school levels. The Teen Pregnancy Unit (TP) was introduced in 1988 as part of the ninth grade health education course. Its five class periods provide information on reproductive biology and teenage pregnancy. Several of the student activities in the Teen Pregnancy unit revolve around the topic of *sexual decision-making*, including discussions and films designed to explore students' abilities to remain abstinent and to resist pressure to have premarital sex.   Since these skills are also congruent with HIV/AIDS prevention, one of the objectives of the present study was to examine the extent to which the Teen Pregnancy Unit may interact synergistically when it is taught before or after the Red Cross HIV/AIDS Prevention Program.

Enhancement 2

Peer Modeling Role Playing Exercises.   As explained earlier, previous preventive intervention research has identified peer modeling and reinforced practice as key approaches to promoting positive self-efficacy beliefs and positive change in health behavior. The American Red Cross Video "A Letter from Brian," presents media models for preventive behaviors and opportunities for vicarious reinforcement for students viewing the video.   We hypothesized that use of a locally produced video depicting Harford County students, coupled with actual in-class demonstrations by the same peer models in the video, would enhance the modeling effects of the American Red Cross video.   Therefore, several role play activities were developed by teachers, students, and research staff to enable students to practice communication and pressure resistance skills.

Three meetings were held with the health teacher at one of the two *enhanced* intervention schools (School 2) to develop the outlines of role play scenarios, the concept of the demonstration video, and instructions for the teachers.   Also, at this time, an acronym (P.R.O.B.E.) was developed to facilitate student practice of communication of specific information through the exercise. The acronym stood for: *P*roblem identification, *R*isk appraisal, *O*ptions for safe problem resolution, *B*ehave preventively, and *E*valuate the consequences.   We have subsequently discovered similarities between the P.R.O.B.E. problem sequence and the S.O.D.A.S. sequence in the Gilchrist, Schinke, Trimble and Cvetkovitch (1987) SLT-based substance abuse prevention curriculum.

Four senior students were recruited from this school by the health teacher to serve as peer models in the demonstration video.

Parental permission was obtained for their participation. It is important to note that because this school already had in place a peer-counseling/role play facilitation team for other subjects (e.g., Students Against Drunk Driving), teens skilled in the use of facilitated role play were already available. The research team, the 4 students, and the health teacher conducted two taping session (90 minutes each) after school. One of the investigators then edited the video. During use in the classroom, teachers usually decided to show portions of the tape highlighting the models developing skills in using P.R.O.B.E. This saved class time for the viewers to practice the modeled skills.

The role-play activities were conducted in the two enhanced intervention schools in the final two days of the five day unit and after the presentation of the core Red Cross HIV/AIDS Prevention Program. Each class was divided into small groups (approximately 4-5 students per group) and students were shown the video with Harford County student models communicating about several locally relevant HIV/AIDS risking scenarios and demonstrating the P.R.O.B.E. sequence. In each classroom, each group of students was given the option of either using a practice scenario already prepared by the project team or developing one of their own. The students that appeared in the demonstration video also facilitated the role playing process among each group's participants. After two days of in-class practice and an evening's homework assignment, the groups performed their role plays either for the teacher alone or in front of the class. (Further details about this activity may be obtained from the authors.)

Enhancement 3

The Photonovel. A photonovel was developed at one site (School 1) to serve as a booster intervention to the AIDS unit. A photonovel is similar to a comic book, but with a storyline that is depicted with photographs of actual students in their social contexts. As in comic books, the dialogue is placed in word bubbles. Students who are involved in the production of the photonovel take part in exploring and applying decision-making skills that may affect their values regarding HIV/AIDS health risks.

Because participants can readily identify with and "own" this HIV/AIDS prevention media, it is hypothesized that they may more readily promote it among their friends and family. In addition, from the standpoint of the student readers, the depiction as well as the active involvement of peers in the photonovel should enhance the *credibility* and the *acceptance* of the health education message, as well as promote increases in readers' *self-efficacy* beliefs, as they observe their peers solving problems within their local environment.

Photonovel development for the present study was coordinated by one of the investigators. It began with a planning meeting with two health education teachers from one of the participating schools to develop a strategy for student recruitment to the production team. Thirteen students from the ninth grade health education classes of this school volunteered to participate. These students were representative of those currently taking health education, and had participated in the Red Cross HIV/AIDS Prevention Program earlier in the semester. At the first student meeting, volunteers were informed about the nature of the project, what their participation would entail and how much they would be compensated. (They were paid a small stipend of about $25 for their participation, which involved approximately 10 sessions after school.) Volunteers were also required to obtain written permission from their parents to participate in this activity.

During the subsequent sessions, the two health teachers at this school and the Coordinating investigator supervised and assisted with all development phases. Work was guided by Rudd, Kichen, & Joslin's, (1980) "How-To Manual for Student Produced Health Education Material." This "How-To" manual details process and production steps, with check lists and summaries to provide planning guides for each phase. It was written by researchers who were actively involved in the production of "Decisions, Decisions," a photonovel developed by ninth grade students of Franklin County Technical School in Massachusetts for the purpose of exploring various situations in which teens felt pressured to smoke.

The photonovel production process included the following steps: (1) students conducted informal interviews with other students

students to gain insights into potential readers' knowledge of HIV/AIDS; (2) they developed a storyline intended to define a conflict and resolution of the conflict; (3) they developed a plot sketch which included the form and structure of the novel; (4) they drew an initial layout with assignments; (5) they gathered photo props and chose actors; (6) they shot the pictures; and (7) they prepared the final layout once screened photos were received from the printer. The final layout was approved by the principal, the County Curriculum Supervisor, and the research team members before it was sent to the printer. The final product was a photonovel entitled "What if ...?". Its 16 pages of storyline contained 23 pictures depicting situations in which teens might risk HIV infection, plus a final page of questions for thought. (A copy of the photonovel and a more detailed instruction sheet, designed to serve as a guide for interested parties, may be obtained from the authors.)

The photonovel was disseminated in the 2nd semester health classes of *School 1* in early June of 1989. First semester students (currently taking physical education) were also asked to attend the second semester health class on that particular day. After reading the photonovel in class, students were asked to answer the questions at the back of the booklet; a class discussion (led by health education instructors) ensued. Photonovel creators were also asked to fill out a short evaluation form before dissemination of the booklet.

INTERVENTION OUTCOME & PROCESS ASSESSMENTS

Assessment Schedule

As outlined in Figure 1, during the 1988-89 academic year, various intervention outcome and process objectives were evaluated at baseline (pre-intervention), immediate post-intervention, and at several short term follow-up intervals (Fall semester = 6 months and Spring semester = 2 months). A longer term follow-up occurred in December of 1989 (1 year for the Fall semester cohort and 8 months for the Spring semester cohort).

Assessment Process and Content

Self-administered, voluntary non-anonymous questionnaires were used on each scheduled assessment occasion. Each student was assigned a unique ID number that allowed linkage of data points. A student's ID number was printed on each survey and his/her name was removed from the cover page as the survey was handed to the student for completion. Before administration of the baseline and each subsequent survey, students were reminded about the nature of the study, and assured about the confidentiality of their responses.

As outlined in Table 3, the questionnaires contained items and scales designed to tap theoretical constructs from the *Health Belief Model* such as perceived threat of AIDS/HIV infection, perceived severity of AIDS, and perceived barriers and benefits to preventive actions (see Table 3, category 4, "Attitudes and Beliefs about HIV/AIDS"). The questionnaire also assessed constructs from Bandura's *Social Learning Theory* model including personal efficacy to prevent AIDS/HIV infection, perceived peer support/pressure, and communication with family and peers (see Table 3 categories 5, 7, 8, and 11). In addition, the baseline survey consisted of items (and categories) pertaining to socioeconomic indicators (1), family and religious values plus present and future aspirations/concerns (2), HIV/AIDS knowledge (3), perceived norms of peer behaviors (10), sexual and dating experience (12, 13), substance use (14), other risk-taking behavior (15), and affective measures such as anxiety and depression (16). The subsequent surveys, that were given pre- and post-administration of each unit (i.e., Teen Pregnancy Unit vs. AIDS Red Cross Prevention Program), and at 2 and 6 month follow-up periods, repeated essential parts of the baseline survey and substituted additional items concerning attitude and behavior changes resulting specifically from the Red Cross and/or Teen Pregnancy curricula. Process evaluations which involved the subjective experiences of students, teachers, and administrators were also conducted at several stages of the project to provide recommendations for refinement of intervention materials and their disseminations.

RESULTS

Due to the scope of variables assessed longitudinally, we have selected to report here the results pertaining to the first three short-term objectives (changes in HIV/AIDS knowledge, communications, and self-efficacy) and to more briefly report on the remaining outcome objectives. A discussion regarding sexual behavior is first provided to inform readers of the potential sexual risk status of youth in this sample. The process evaluation variables reported here involve parent and teacher acceptance of the HIV/AIDS prevention evaluation project, as well as student ratings of the two enhanced intervention components: the peer modeling/role play and the photonovel.

Outcome Objectives

Pre-Intervention Sexual Behavior. Baseline and subsequent changes in the onset of sexual intercourse, frequency of sexual activity and precautions taken during sex are important variables for general population HIV/AIDS prevention programming. As seen in Table 4, 33.8% of 1st semester students and 40.1% of 2nd semester students reported being sexually active at their respective baselines. Of those sexually active, approximately the same proportion (30.7% of 1st semester students and 28.8% of 2nd semester students) reported having more than 3 partners in their lifetime. Similarly, 20.8% of 1st semester students and 24.7% of 2nd semester students reported beginning sexual intercourse at or before 13 years of age. With regard to condom use, 63% of students both semesters reported using a condom at last intercourse. Table 5 shows school differences for baseline sexualbehavior. Only in the second semester cohort were there any pre-intervention significant school differences for the percent sexually active an for the mean number of sexual partners reported.

Second semester students (only) were asked at baseline about recent behavioral changes due to concern about HIV/AIDS. About 25% (105/428) responded "Yes" that they had already changed their behavior in the past year. Of these students, 27.7% reported using condoms, 14.3% reported being more selective in their choice of partners, and 7.6% reported saying "No" to sex when pressured by a date.

Post Intervention Sexual Behavior

Open ended questions dealing with behavioral change were asked at immediate posttest and subsequent follow-ups both first and second semesters. Second semester students were asked whether participating in the HIV/AIDS curriculum had lead them to form intentions to change behavior and/or to adopt actual behavior changes that would reduce risk for HIV exposure. Eight month follow-up data from the second semester cohort indicated an intervention effect. Specifically, there was a significant linear trend for intentions to change behavior involving sexual transmission risks. Compared to students who only received the core RC AIDS Prevention Program, students who received one or both of the enhanced interventions were increasingly more likely to report that they intended to change their behaviors (X^2=5.78, df=1, p=.016). More detail about these findings are reported elsewhere (Platt, Baldwin, Rolf, Perry, Alexander & Pankey, 1990). Future analyses will focus on these sexual behavior related variables as a function of efficacy beliefs, other types of risk behavior, gender and other individual difference variables.

KNOWLEDGE ABOUT HIV/AIDS

One of the objectives of the Red Cross HIV/AIDS Prevention Program for Youth has always been to increase youth's knowledge about HIV/AIDS. Table 6 lists the questions that were asked regarding HIV/AIDS knowledge. A knowledge scale score was calculated for each student by scoring each correctly answered question as 1 point. Sixteen items were repeated on both baseline and immediate posttest questionnaires for both first and second semesters. Given that many of the 16 items were almost always answered correctly, a briefer representative subset of 5 items was selected for follow-up assessments at 6 months (1st semester) and 2 months (2nd semester).

HIV/AIDS Knowledge at Baseline

Because there were no significant differences in baseline knowledge scores by semester, many of the analyses presented here used data that were combined from both semesters. (It is important to note, however, that within the same semester, there were significant school differences in baseline knowledge scores, e.g., for second semester, Kruskai-Wallis test; $X^2=20.61$, $df=1$, $p<.001$). As seen in Table 6, for the 16-item knowledge scale, the mean score for all students at baseline was 14.04 items correct (range=0-16; SD=2.21); at immediate posttest the mean increased to 15.22 items correct (SD=1.55). For the 5-item knowledge scale, the mean score for all students (semesters combined) at baseline was 4.07 items correct, (range=0.5; SD=.955); in subsequent follow-ups the means increased to 4.61 items correct (SD=7.27) at immediate posttest and 4.45 items correct (SD=1.02) at 2 and 6 month follow-up.

Evidence for Intervention Effects on HIV/AIDS Knowledge at Immediate Posttest

Across both semesters, 23.5% of the students (N=173/736) had perfect baseline scores on the 16 item knowledge scale. Of the remaining 563 students, 76.0% improved their score immediately following the Red Cross HIV/AIDS Prevention Program, and at that time, 57.7% (431/712) achieved perfect scores. Because preliminary ANCOVA's demonstrated significant interactions between baseline scores and school, each school was examined separately for changes due to the interventions. These paired t-tests revealed that the students in each school setting demonstrated statistically significant increases in knowledge at immediate posttest after the RC program (all t's $\geq$ 2.29, p<.001).

Analysis of immediate posttest scores comparing students of enhanced vs. nonenhanced intervention schools (i.e., with the former having the peer modeling/role play) demonstrated no significant differences. This suggests that the role playing exercise had little additional impact beyond the Red Cross HIV/AIDS Prevention Program on the general knowledge score.

HIV/AIDS Knowledge at Follow-up

The 5-item subset of the 16-item knowledge score was included at 2 and 6 month follow-up to assess longer term effects. About 38% (N=277/733) answered all 5 questions correctly at baseline and at immediate posttest. Subsequently, 75% of those who had not achieved a perfect score at baseline (N=324/433) increased their score at immediate posttest, so that 65% (283/433) of them were answering all 5 items correctly. Longer term follow-up showed negligible decay in knowledge scores, as only 11.9% (80/675) scored less than their baseline level, and in total, 67.8% answered all 5 questions correctly at this time. No significant differences in decay of knowledge were seen across semesters (X^2=6.74, df=5, p=0.240), despite the differing intervals between baseline and either 2 month or 6 month follow-up.

There was also no significant difference (either semester) in scores achieved by students at School 1 which was the only school to receive the photonovel, compared to students of the other schools. This suggests the photonovel did *not* produce a "booster" effect for HIV/AIDS knowledge.

MISCONCEPTIONS ABOUT HIV/AIDS TRANSMISSION

For 2nd Semester students only, we identified six items most often answered incorrectly (i.e., items missed by more than 15% of the students). As seen in Table 6, these misconceptions (superscripted 3) included risk of acquiring HIV infection through casual contact. From these items, we created an HIV/AIDS Misconception scale score, where each student was assigned one point for each item they answered *correctly* (thus a score of "0" reflected *incorrect* answers on all 6 items). As with the General Knowledge scale score, there were baseline differences between schools (Kruskal-Wallis tests; X^2=26.86, df=1, p<.001).

Intervention Effects on Misconceptions

The pattern of HIV/AIDS misconception scores is shown in Figure 3. Only nine percent (39/435) of the 2nd semester students correctly identified all 6 misconceptions as *untrue* on the baseline questionnaire. Subsequently at immediate posttest, 84.9% of the remaining 371 students increased their scores. Overall, at immediate posttest 59% (242/410) correctly identified as *untrue* all six misconceptions. Paired t-test comparisons for each school demonstrated that students' misconceptions decreased significantly across all schools (all t's $\geq$ 10.26, p<.001). Further, at subsequent follow-up, (2 months later), 53% of the students (221/412) retained the maximum score of 6. There were no significant differences between students of enhanced vs. nonenhanced intervention schools at immediate posttest or 2 month follow-up, adjusting for baseline levels with ANCOVA.

SELF-EFFICACY BELIEFS REGARDING HIV/AIDS PREVENTIVE BEHAVIORS

As shown in Table 7, we asked 1st and 2nd Semester students how confident they were about their ability to accomplish different tasks relevant to HIV/AIDS prevention. For each item, they self-rated themselves on a 10-step, 100-point scale ranging from "Definitely Cannot Do It" to "Definitely Can Do It." Because of the different sequencing of the curricula 1st versus 2nd semester (i.e., 1st=TP-RC; 2nd=RC-TP), only the appropriate self-efficacy items were asked at each assessment. In addition, based on 1st semester process data, one item was added and one item was modified 2nd semester (as compared to 1st semester). Thus, because not all items remained comparable between first and second semesters, analyses of self-efficacy variables were conducted separately for the two semesters. Since the RC AIDS Prevention Program was taught before the Teen Pregnancy Unit during the 2nd semester and, because the enhanced interventions were introduced at that time, this chapter reports only on self-efficacy data from the second semester cohort.

The ten self-efficacy items in the baseline survey were

subjected to principal components factor analysis with varimax rotation. This produced three factors as observed in Table 7. The factors can serve as scales which are fairly robust with Cronbach alpha's ranging from .73 to .80. These scales appear to denote three domains of AIDS-related self-efficacy beliefs: Sexual Pressure Resistance Skills (or Negative Assertion), HIV/AIDS Prevention Communication Skills, and Positive Assertion Skills.

Self-Efficacy at Baseline

ANOVAs revealed that there were significant differences between males and females for each scale ($F's \geq$ 18.00, df=1, p<.001), with females reporting significantly higher efficacy. These gender differences are shown in Figure 4. In addition, at baseline, the adolescents who reported still being virgins also reported significantly more self-efficacy regarding ability to resist sexual pressure (Scale 1) compared to their sexually active classmates, $F(1,418)$=19.47, p<.001.

Intervention Effects on Self-Efficacy

Overall, mean scores for all three scales of self-efficacy (2nd semester) increased from baseline to immediate posttest and from baseline to 2 month follow-up for males and females of *all* schools. As seen in Table 8, using paired t-test analyses, the only positive shifts in self-efficacy scores which were *not* significant (at p<.05) at *immediate posttest* included: boy's efficacy in sexual pressure resistance skills and communication skills, and girl's efficacy in positive assertion skills.

Enhanced Intervention Effects

There was also evidence to suggest that the enhanced interventions may have increased self-efficacy beliefs above the standard Red Cross HIV/AIDS Prevention Program. For example, at School 1, boys who experienced the role playing showed significantly higher confidence in their HIV/AIDS preventive communication skills immediately following the AIDS unit than boys at the comparison school who did not participate in the role playing activity, controlling for baseline levels (ANCOVA F=4.84, p=.030). There was also a trend for girls at School 1 to report higher communication efficacy than girls at School 3 at immediate posttest (ANCOVA F=2.09, p=.15).

Subgroup Patterns in Self-Efficacy Changes

To explore the direction of change, we created a 3-level categorical change score for each self-efficacy scale, indicating negative change, positive change or no change.[1] As seen in Figure 5, for sexual pressure resistance skills, females at one of the enhanced intervention schools (School 1) demonstrated significantly more change in the positive direction than females at the nonenhanced comparison School (X^2=9.17, df=2, p=.01).

Changes in self-efficacy were also found to be related to level of sexual experience such as *virgin vs. nonvirgin status*. For example, in another report (Baldwin et al., 1989), we described how sexually experienced students vs. virgins showed proportionally more positive change for *sexual pressure resistance skills* (X^2=6.54, df=2, p=.038). Also, for *positive assertion skills*, as compared to those who reported being sexually active (X^2=12.33, df=2, p=.002). These findings suggest that the curriculum had differential effects for sexually experienced vs. less experienced students. We are presently pursuing further analyses to examine these relationships.

COMMUNICATION ABOUT HIV/AIDS

Student-Parent Communication

The American Red Cross HIV/AIDS Prevention Program for Youth was also designed to increase student's ability to discuss HIV/AIDS with their parents and with other students. We asked participants if they had talked to one of their parents about AIDS and/or related topics before and after the HIV/AIDS curriculum.

In order to highlight an expected intervention effect, the time frame in which the question was asked was shifted from the *previous* month at baseline to the *previous week* at immediate posttest and at follow-up. Baseline, immediate posttest and follow-up rates for student-parent discussion topics are presented in Table 9. At baseline, 46.5% of 1st semester students and 33.8% of 2nd semester students had talked to one of their parents about AIDS during the past month.

As observed in Table 9, the curriculum had a positive impact on student-parent communication regarding HIV/AIDS. Figure 6 also demonstrates that the percent of students who reported talking to one of their parents about AIDS increased across all schools 2nd Semester after the intervention, and a very similar positive trend was seen for 1st semester students. Overall, there was a nearly 20% increase in student-parent HIV/AIDS communications for students of all schools from baseline to immediate posttest.

Enhancement Effects on HIV/AIDS Communications with Parents

Figure 6 illustrates that students who received the enhanced intervention reported greater communication with their parents at immediate posttest than students of their respective comparison schools. Students of School 1 (one of the enhanced intervention schools) showed significantly more communication than students of its comparison school (School 3) at immediate posttest (X^2=5.79, df=1, p=.05) and at 2-month follow-up (X^2=5.07, df=1, p=.02). We believe that this sustained communication (at 2-month follow-up) may have been due to the booster effect of the photonovel, which was distributed one week before the administration of the 2-month follow-up survey.

Curriculum Sequence Effect on HIV/AIDS Communication with Parents

There was also evidence to suggest that teaching the Teen Pregnancy Unit before the RC AIDS Program enhanced student-parent communication about sex, in general. For example, at one school, significantly more students 1st semester reported talking to their parents about sex after the TP-RC sequence compared to 2nd semester students in the same school was were evaluated after taking the RC AIDS Program and before participating in the Teen Pregnancy Unit (X^2=12.72, df=1, p=.0017).

Student-Student Communication About HIV/AIDS at Baseline

Students were asked at each assessment whether they had ever talked to any person their own age about HIV/AIDS prevention and several other topics. They were also asked *how many* people their own age they had talked to about HIV/AIDS. At baseline, no time interval was specified for past communications; however, "during the *past week*" was the interval specified at immediate posttest and at both follow-ups. At baseline, 35.4% of *all* students (259/731) answered "Yes" to the questions, "Have you ever talked with any persons your own age about how to prevent AIDS?" There was a significant difference at baseline between schools, with students of School 4 (both semesters) and students of School 3 (second semester) reporting fewer "Yes" responses; (1st semester: X^2=6.25, df=2, p=0.044, 2nd semester: X^2=9.87, df=3, p=0.019). In addition, there was a gender difference with girls communicating more with fellow students.

Table 10 summarizes baseline and intervention findings by semester. At baseline, students indicated that the *number of peers* each had talked to ranged from 1 to 50, with 15.6% of 1st semester students and 9.9% of 2nd semester students reporting talking with 4 or more people. There were no significant differences by school, gender, or race.

Intervention Effects on Student-Student HIV/AIDS Communication

At immediate posttest for both semesters combined, 42.9% of *all* students (301/701) answered "Yes" that they had talked to their peers about AIDS in the *past week*. However, there was a significant difference by semester, with the first semester students reporting talking more ($X^2=6.22$, $df=1$, $p<.01$). This variable was therefore analyzed separately for each semester. Overall, at immediate posttest, 52.3% of first semester students replied "Yes" to this question, representing a significant increase in communication with peers immediately following the AIDS Unit (McNemar $X^2=34.3$, $df=1$, $p<.001$). Further, there were no significant differences by school, race, or gender. For 2nd semester at immediate posttest, there was a significant difference across schools, with students of Schools 1 and 2 (the enhanced intervention schools), reporting significantly more "Yes" replies ($X^2=25.04$, $df=3$, $p<.001$). There was also a significant difference by gender, with more females reporting that they had talked with other students about AIDS prevention ($X^2=14.04$, $df=1$, $p=0.0002$).

With regard to the *number* of peers that students reported talking to about AIDS prevention, McNemar chi-square analyses demonstrated a significant pre- to post-test increase in the proportion of students talking to 4 or more peers immediately after the AIDS curriculum (McNemar $X^2 \geq 4.6$, $p<.05$). Students who responded to this question said they talked to between 1 to 50 peers with 21.4% of 1st semester students and 19.3% of 2nd semester students reporting talking to 4 or more people. There were no differences by gender, race or school, suggesting that the effect of the role play was to encourage communication in general rather than to influence the actual *number* of peers students had talked to.

Student-Student Communications at Follow-up

With regard to longer term follow-up (e.g., 6 months post AIDS Unit), 11.8% of 1st semester students responded "Yes" that they had spoken to their peers about AIDS during the previous *week*. This indicates a significant decrease (McNemar $X^2 \geq 36.9$, $p<.001$). There were no significant differences by race, gender or *school* including School 1 students who received the photonovel in the week prior to the follow-up questionnaire. In the 1st semester, thirty students responded to the question asking about the *number of peers* they had spoken with, and they reported a range of numbers between 1 and 33, with 6.5% reporting talking with 4 or more people. These findings suggest that HIV/AIDS peer to peer communication increased during the unit, remained very high for several weeks, then declined over subsequent months.

At 2 month follow-up for 2nd semester students, 13.8% responded "Yes" to the question about any HIV/AIDS prevention communication with peers during the past week. At this shorter term follow-up (2 vs. 6 months), there was a significant decrease from previous levels of communication (McNemar $X^2=62.9$, $p<.001$). However, a significant difference was seen across schools. Students of School 1, who had received the photonovel just prior to the follow-up, reported significantly more "Yes" responses than the students of other schools ($X^2=14.33$, $df=3$, $p=0.003$). There were no differences by gender. Students who responded to the question about the number of peers they had spoken to reported a range of numbers between 1 and 54, with 6.0% reporting talking to 4 or more people. There was no significant conclusion that although peer to peer HIV/AIDS communication was stimulated by the enhanced interventions, the effect was to increase communication in general, rather than to influence the actual *number* of peers with whom they talked.

PROCESS EVALUATION RESULTS

Appreciation for the Programs and Materials

Both 1st and 2nd semester students were asked a series of questions regarding the Red Cross workbook and video, the role playing exercises, and the photonovel, at 6 and 2 month follow-ups, respectively. Overall, the American Red Cross HIV/AIDS Prevention Program for Youth and the supplemental intervention enhancements were very well received by both students and teachers. In brief, 1st and 2nd semesters students, respectively: (1) judged the quality of the Red Cross (RC) workbook and video to be *"better"* (50%, 47%) *than the other materials used in their health education classes*; (2) said these materials "very much" (56%, 52%) or "somewhat" (34%, 38%) *helped them to accept responsibilities for AIDS prevention*; (3) reported the RC materials "very much" (59%, 57%) or "somewhat" (32%, 31%) *helped them avoid AIDS-risking behaviors*; and (4) said the RC materials "very much" (51%, 47%) or "somewhat" *helped them to know more about AIDS*. Further details of student acceptance of the RC printed and video materials can be found in Pankey, Baldwen, Rolf, Platt, Perry, and Alexander (1990).

Role Playing Activities

In their responses to the three open-ended questions (regarding most liked aspects, least liked aspects and suggestions for improvement), students generally rated the role playing activity positively. The majority of students liked the chance to work in groups and to have the opportunity to openly discuss feelings about AIDS and related topics among their *peers*. They also liked writing the scripts and portraying different characters in the skits who were confronted with different HIV-risking scenarios. Most students said they wished they had had more opportunities to practice their role plays. Least liked aspects were the potential for embarrassment and having to get up in front of the class to perform their original role play (required by one teacher). The most frequent suggestions for improvement were allowing more time for development of role plays and providing more examples.

Students were also asked at 2 month follow-up if they practiced role-playing with: (1) a person in their health class, (2) a person not in their health class, (3) a boyfriend or girlfriend, (4) a family member. The majority (83%) reported practicing the role plays with someone in their health class (as the activity was intended), while fewer (13.9%) reported practicing the role plays with someone outside of their class, a boyfriend/girlfriend (14.3%) or a family member (10.3%). Interestingly, significantly more males than females said they had practiced role playing with a date (X^2=4.8, df=1, p=.028). Students also rated the degree to which the role-playing exercises helped them to communicate about pregnancy prevention, AIDS prevention, and assisting a friend to solve personal problems. Overall, the ratings were positive with only a fifth (20% or less) reporting that the role plays had *no* influence at all on helping them to communicate about these topics.

Student Appraisals of the Photonovel

The thirteen student volunteers who created the photonovel spoke very highly about the group planning and production processes, emphasizing the cooperation generated among participants, meeting new friends, and having an opportunity to teach others about sexual risks. In addition, in the process evaluation portion of the follow-up surveys, all the students who read the photonovel reported that they enjoyed reading it as a classroom activity. Overall, 78.8% of the students thought the booklet was "fun to read," 73.6% thought the characters seemed real and 84% thought the HIV/AIDS risk situations depicted in the photonovel seemed real. Students were asked whether or not they thought the booklet would help them to make some decisions about having sexual intercourse, and the majority answered affirmatively (67.8% of 1st semester students shown the photonovel two weeks before the 6 month follow-up assessment and 55.4% of 2nd semester students who read the photonovel 2 months after the RC unit).

DISCUSSION

Success in Achieving the Project Objectives

Increasing HIV/AIDS Knowledge in 80% of Students. Although initial knowledge about HIV/AIDS was high at baseline, our findings indicate that the American Red Cross HIV/AIDS Prevention Program for Youth produced significant and lasting increases in general HIV/AIDS knowledge among students of both semesters. For the 16-items general knowledge score, 76% of all students who had not achieved a perfect score at baseline *improved* their score at immediate posttest. The program also produced significant decreases in HIV/AIDS misconceptions which were assessed among students of the second semester cohort; 84.9% of those who did not have a perfect score at baseline reported fewer misconceptions at immediate posttest. The role playing and photonovel activities appeared to have no additional impact on knowledge. The importance of other variables on AIDS knowledge scores (e.g., SES, academic skill as measured by G.P.A.) remains to be explored in future multivariate analyses.

Increasing Relevant Health Promotion Efficacy Beliefs in 70% of Students. In general, self-efficacy beliefs regarding HIV/AIDS preventive behaviors increased among students at *all* schools after the interventions. During 2nd semester, students' efficacy beliefs increased as much as 50%. Our findings lend some evidence to suggest that supplementing the Red Cross HIV/AIDS Prevention Program for Youth with activities such as role-playing and the photonovel strengthened feelings of confidence for some individuals, as there were instances where students of the enhanced intervention school demonstrated significantly higher efficacy scores than students of their respective comparison schools at posttest. We have reconsidered, however, the appropriateness of our initial prediction that all participates should demonstrate increases in self-efficacy. It now seems unreasonable to expect that *everyone* should show such increases in efficacy after interventions which provide practice of relevant skills. For example, some sexually inexperienced adolescents may initially *overestimate* their ability to communicate with others about these topics, and subsequently give more realistic and somewhat lower self-ratings when they discover how difficult it can actually be when they try practicing the role plays. We now expect our interventions to interact with individual differences and contextual situations. Further analyses are underway and are indicating how subgroups of youth responded more favorably (in terms of changes in self-efficacy) to the mass targeted RC AIDS Prevention Program. In addition, we are finding how subgroup differences (based on baseline efficacy and sexual experience) result in differential change among those who received the role play enhancement.

Increasing Communication in 50% of the Students

The Red Cross HIV/AIDS Prevention Program for Youth also appeared to have a positive impact on *both* student-student communication and student-parent communication regarding HIV/AIDS. At baseline, 35.4% of all students reported *ever* talking to a friend about AIDS; at immediate posttest, 42.9% said they had talked to a friend within the *past week*. During 2nd semester, students of the enhanced intervention schools reported more conversation with peers about HIV/AIDS prevention both immediately after the unit and two months later, compared to students who received only the core RC program.

Overall, there was a 20% increase in student-parent communication about HIV/AIDS from baseline to immediate posttest. Students of the enhanced intervention schools demonstrated greater communication than students of their respective comparison schools at immediate post-test and 2 month follow-up. There was also some evidence to suggest: (1) that the photonovel served as an effective booster intervention, especially with regard to the follow-up findings of increased student-parent communication about HIV/AIDS 2 months after the unit; and (2) that teaching the Teen Pregnancy Unit before the AIDS unit enhanced student-parent communication about sex.

It is important to point out that these increases in student-parent communications did not produce complaints to principals or health education teachers about the content of the curriculum or the process of evaluation. This is a strong indication of the readiness of Harford County parents to accept the evaluation of the Red Cross HIV/AIDS Prevention Program and the enhancement of HIV/AIDS prevention curricula. We believe that the school system's reputation for commitment to health education and the careful informed consent procedures employed for the present project contributed to parental acceptance. We also think that the curriculum's effort to communicate and evaluate widely held values about the family's role in health promotion may have fostered parental trust.

Other Outcome Objectives

We are pursuing a more extensive examination of the correlates and apparent temporal sequences leading to changes in sexual behavior and other cognitive and behavioral variables relevant to HIV/AIDS prevention. The shorter term and longer term follow-up data have provided intriguing preliminary results. One example concerns the transition from virgin to non-virgin status. In all, about 80 students reported becoming non-virgins during the year long series of assessments. During each interval, the variables predictive of change included expected age of first intercourse, current risk-taking, perceptions of peer pressure to have sex, substance use, sexual activity of close friends and self-efficacy beliefs concerning ability to resist pressure to have sex. Experience with alcohol and illicit substances were also predictive of outcome status. In discriminant function analyses, the number of different drugs ever tried correctly classified about 60% of those remaining virgins and 85% of those changing. Using all variables described above plus the number of substances tried predicted up to 81% of those remaining virgins and up to 87% of those converting (Platt, Rolf, Baldwin, Perry, Alexander & Pankey, 1990).

STRENGTHS AND LIMITATIONS OF THE RESEARCH PROJECT

Study Design

There were some important strengths to the design which include the following points: (1) given the approximate split-half nature of assignment by semester to the required health education class, we were able to replicate most aspects of the evaluation of the HIV/AIDS interventions both within schools across semesters and across school sites; (2) the sample sizes were large representing over 90% of all 9th-grade students; (3) our assessment schedule provided ample longitudinal information on continuity and change in individual differences and on short term and longer term intervention effects. We also recognize the design limitations of this study, especially with regard to the use of non-equivalent contrast schools and the fact that the RC program was embedded in a semester-long health education class. Random assignment of schools to intervention and non-intervention conditions was not feasible because non-intervention schools were unavailable (the curriculum was required for all ninth graders by the County). We did attempt to match comparison schools based on similarities in basic sociodemographics; however, a few within pair differences were observed on our planned outcome variables at baseline. We have attempted to control for some of these differences through analysis of covariance and other statistical techniques. However, it remains difficult to be entirely certain that other meditating factors may not have had an effect (e.g., subtle differences among teachers' implementation of the curriculum).

Further, *random assignment* to 1st and 2nd semester cohorts by the evaluation team was not possible as the schools had established the class schedules during the previous summer vacation. However, sample bias is negligible given that we achieved a near total sample of all ninth graders and have found semester cohorts to be very similar. It has become very apparent that using the "school" as the unit of analysis may not always be appropriate, in that within each school there is a very heterogenous mix of students. We believe that to assess the effects of these interventions more accurately one needs to identify subgroups of youth based upon relevant individual difference variables (e.g., risk-taking versus cautious youth, multiproblem versus typical youth) and examine how these different groups of students responded to the interventions both within and across schools.

Limitations of Self-Report Data from Adolescents

In dealing with self-reported behavior, there is always the concern that the responses are not entirely truthful. This is a special concern when self-reports (e.g., regarding sexual intercourse) cannot be checked against objective behaviors. Therefore, we employed several means of attempting to ensure that we obtained truthful and reliable responses. First, before administering the questionnaires to the students, the students were reassured about the confidentiality of their responses as well as the importance of the study in helping to develop new HIV/AIDS educational programs for youth in Harford County Schools. Secondly, specific topics considered likely candidates for distortions (e.g., sexual behavior) were repeated in different parts of the same questionnaire to obtain some measure of consistency of responses. In instances where questionnaires were suspect (less than 3% on the most suspect variables), the entire case was excluded from analyses. Further, if information on sexual behavior (i.e., virginity status, age of first intercourse, number of sexual partners, and total number of sexual acts) changed unrealistically between baseline and follow-up, a discrepancy was noted for that case.

Consistency checks of response levels and patterns within subject, and across schools and semesters revealed, that with very few exceptions, students *did* answer consistently, and baseline subsamples produced highly similar responses. Further, the data on sexual behavior seemed reasonable in light of other studies. For example, the prevalence of sexually active ninth graders in Harford County (33.8%, 1st semester; 40.1%, 2nd semester) were similar to reports by Alexander, Ensminger, Kim, Smith, Johnson, and Dolan (1989) for a comparable large multi-school sample of slightly younger students from three rural counties on the Chesapeake's Eastern Shore. In the Alexander et al. (1989) study, 39.8% of White eighth graders reported being sexually active.

Variation in Curriculum Implementation

By using the acting health education teachers of the school system, we could not expect to precisely control the teaching of the curriculum. We did attempt to lace restrictions on teachers in terms of what and how much information they presented during this five day unit, but it was difficult to completely control their actions. Process data revealed some variability among the eight instructors who taught the curriculum in the five high schools during the two semesters. Most notably, the actual sequence of RC activities varied, some teachers provided extra credit opportunities and additional homework assignments, and some instructors graded activities while others did not. This lack of process control adds some unmeasured bias to the results. However, from a pragmatic perspective, it is important to view the project's positive outcomes as evidence for the robustness and flexibility of the Red Cross HIV/AIDS Prevention Program and its viability in heterogeneous sets of teacher-led classrooms.

CONCLUSIONS AND RECOMMENDATIONS

The present study has provided substantial evidence that an HIV/AIDS education curriculum can produce important positive effects among ninth graders in Harford County, Maryland. Our results also point to the existence of important subgroup differences. Mass targeted school-based HIV/AIDS preventive interventions should prove generally beneficial, but they will likely have some different effects on students as a function of both individual differences and contextual (environmental) factors. Therefore, we recommend that HIV/AIDS education programs be adapted to meet the needs of different subgroups of teens who are embedded in different school and community environments. In schools with identifiable groups of higher risk adolescents (e.g., teen parents), more explicit and extensive HIV/AIDS prevention skills training should be added. For example, both videos ("Don't Forget Sherrie" and "A Letter From Brian") might be shown when applying the Red Cross Program in a school which has an equal number of white and black students. (This was indeed one of the recommendations of students from School 5 in the present study.)

We also believe that HIV/AIDS curricula should be incorporated into comprehensive school health programs that provide students with a *series* of opportunities and contexts in which to practice HIV/AIDS prevention communication skills. We found, for example, that the Teen Pregnancy Unit primed students for the AIDS unit in terms of acquainting them with basic information about relevant anatomy and physiology, and probably setting the stage for more in-depth discussion of sexual behavior as it applies to risks for HIV infection. The Harford County Public School System provides an exemplary health education curriculum which includes a comprehensive range of prevention units designed for teens: (e.g., units on teenage pregnancy, AIDS, sexually transmitted diseases, drugs, accident prevention, etc.). We believe that it is important to *reinforce* consistent practice of prevention skills, including communication of prevention messages, across these various units.

As other researchers have noted (e.g., DiClemente, 1989; Flora & Thoresen, 1989; Hingson, Strunin, Berlin & Heeren, 1990), HIV/AIDS curricula that just relay facts are outdated. Most students have already been exposed to factual information about HIV/AIDS from a variety of sources. Certainly, information about AIDS is essential to improving decision-making skills, but today and in the near future, emphasis should be placed on correcting misconceptions about HIV transmission and improving personal risk assessment. It also appears that providing HIV/AIDS prevention information and skill development activities does not exhaust personal interest in learning *more* about AIDS. Our evaluation objective was to demonstrate that 60% or more of the students would express motivation to learn more about HIV prevention. After the AIDS intervention, 84% still wanted more information about HIV/AIDS. Therefore, additional sources of information should be made available and/or follow-up (booster) sessions on key issues should be integrated into subsequent curriculum units in the same or related courses.

With regard to our two experimental enhancements to the Red Cross Program, we have the following recommendations. The role play exercise is a low cost, low labor intensive activity which generates a great deal of student and teacher participation and positive response. It opens up otherwise difficult topics for discussion and practical applications of HIV/AIDS knowledge and prevention skills. Role play (including scenario development) creates a relatively safe environment for discussion and application. Our project's role play exercise could be improved in its demonstration video and structuring of student activities. As implemented, it did not always result in the practice of a broad range of communication skills due to students focusing on some aspect of a scenario that could not be realistically addressed in class. Given that reinforced practice is a key element for most successful programs of behavior change, the role play exercise did provide many more opportunities for the teens to discuss important issues, than occurred in classes which did not use the exercise.

In addition, a video can be a useful ice-breaker for initiating the role play activities. It is not necessary if trained peer facilitators appear in person. However, if a video is developed, for efficiency or reliability purposes it should not be longer than 8 to 10 minutes or insufficient class time will remain to allow development of student dialogues. If peer facilitators are to be used, they should have already received instruction from the curriculum, have a sound knowledge of the project's HIV/AIDS prevention objectives and they should be well rehearsed in the role play exercise. Our project would have benefitted from more time for the practice of the role plays (i.e., more than three hours) and more student input into the development of a useable portfolio of student developed scenarios.

The photonovel, while very positively received, can be a labor intensive project. It can also be too costly for broadscale implementation. (In our study, the total cost was $1900 which included the payment of teachers ($875) and students ($350) and printing costs ($600) for 500 copies of the 16-page booklet.) The costs for implementing this activity could be greatly reduced through various creative approaches. Some suggestions include: (1) integrating the development of the photonovel into a photojournalism class or the school newspaper; (2) meeting at times when the teacher(s) would not require overtime payment; and (3) eliminating stipends for the students by using some other type of incentive (e.g., extra credit).

In summary, HIV/AIDS prevention curricula for youth must go beyond simply conveying facts. More creative and subgroup specific strategies should be developed that involve the intended audiences in planning, testing, and even disseminating the messages. Efforts that incorporate age-appropriate skills-training (e.g., developing resistance skills, behavior rehearsal, social modeling with performance feedback) may prove very useful in helping some youth achieve behavior change. Further, for some teens, the classroom and the school can be effective channels for influencing their behavior. We believe that the types of interventions developed in this study offer much promise with respect to the ability to modify adolescents' sexual attitudes and behavior. We would strongly urge others to pursue the application and evaluation of these types of theory-based strategies in the much needed effort to diminish the spread of HIV/AIDS to the youth of this country.

Acknowledgments

The authors wish to acknowledge the Harford County Public School System's collaborative spirit and dedication to fully implementing this evaluation research project. We are grateful for the guidance provided by Ed Saunders, Supervisor of Curriculum, and Jack McCracken, Supervisor of Health and High School Physical Education of Harford County, Maryland. Five high school principals, health education teachers, and students made the experimental interventions and the non-anonymous longitudinal data collection possible. Key personnel at each high school included: *C. Milton Wright High School* - Mr. Robert Garbacik (Principal), Mr. Charles Jensen (Health teacher), Mr. Richard Greene (Health teacher); *Joppatown High School* - Mr. F. Thomas

Pomilla (Asst. Principal), Ms. Barbara Day (Health teacher); *Fallston High School* - Mr. Frank Stultz (Principal), Mr. Mark Puckett (Health teacher); *Edgewood High School*- Mr. Carol Roberts (Principal), Mrs. Kay Kleman (Health teacher), Ms. Lin Van Name (Health teacher); *Aberdeen High School* - Dr. Thomas Dubel (Principal), Mr. Richard Slutzky (Health teacher), Ms. Dawn Rathgeber (Health teacher).

NOTE

[1]A fairly stringent criteria was used to measure "change." An individual's *mean* score had to increase or decrease more than 10 points from his/her original score to be considered positive or negative change, respectively. In addition, only those students with scores less than 100% at both time points were included in these analyses.

REFERENCES

AIDS Administration, Division of AIDS Surveillance. (January 31, 1990). Maryland AIDS Update.

Alexander, C., Ensminger, M., Kim, Y., Smith, J., Johnson, K., & Dolan, L. (1989). Early sexual activity among adolescents in small towns and rural areas: Race and gender patterns. *Family Planning Perspectives, 21(6),* 261-266.

Alexander, C., Kim, Y., Ensminger, M., Johnson, K., Smith, J., & Dolan, L. (In press). A measure of risk-taking for young adolescents: Reliability and validity assessments. *Journal of Youth and Adolescence.*

Baldwin, J., Rolf, J., Pankey, J., Alexander, C., Fowler, M., Petty, M., & Platt, M. (1989). *Evaluation of AIDS prevention programs for rural and suburban adolescents.* A paper presented at the American Public Health Association Conference in Chicago, October, 23.

Bandura, A. (1986a). *Social foundations of thought and action.* Englewood Cliffs, NJ: Prentice-Hall.

Bandura, A. (1986b). Self-efficacy mechanism in physiological activation and health promoting behavior. In J. Madden IV, S. Matthysse & J. Barchas (Eds.), *Adaptation, learning and affect.* New York: Raven Press.

Botvin, G.J. (1986). Substance abuse prevention research: Recent developments and future directions. *Journal of School Health, 56,* 369-374.

Brooks-Gunn, J., Boyer, C.B., & Hein, K. (1988, November). Preventing HIV infection and AIDS in children and adolescents. Behavioral research and intervention strategies. *American Psychologist, 43(11),* 958-964.

Brooks-Gunn, J., & Furstenberg, F.F., Jr. (1989). Adolescent sexual behavior. *American Psychologist, 44(2),* 249-257.

Brown, L.K., Fritz, G.K., & Barone, V.J. (1989). The impact of AIDS education on junior and senior high school students: A pilot study. *Journal of Adolescent Health Care, 10,* 386-392.

Buhrmester, D., Furman, W., Wittenberg, M.T., & Reis, H.T. (1988). Five domains of interpersonal competence in peer relationships. *Journal of Personality and Social Psychology, 55(6),* 991-1008.

Centers for Disease Control (1990). *HIV/AIDS Weekly Surveillance Report,* January 1990.

Clark, S., Zabin, L., & Hardy, J. (1984). Sex, contraception, and parenthood: Experience and attitudes among urban Black young men. *Family Planning Perspectives, 16* (Mach/April), 77-82.

DiClemente, R.J. (1989). Prevention of Human Immunodeficiency Virus Infection among adolescents: The interplay of health education and public policy in the development and implementation of school-based AIDS education programs. *AIDS Education and Prevention, 1(1),* 70-78.

DiClemente, R.J., Boyer, C.B., & Morales, E.W. (1988). Minorities and AIDS: Knowledge, attitudes, and misconceptions among black and latino adolescents. *American Journal of Public Health, 78,* 55-57.

DiClemente, R.J., Pies, C., Stoller, E. et al. (1989). Evaluation of school-based AIDS education curricula in San Francisco. *Journal of Sex Research, 26(2),* 188-198.

DiClemente, R.J., Zorn, J., & Temoshok, L. (1987). The association of gender, ethnicity, and length of residence in the Bay area to adolescents' knowledge and attitudes about acquired immune deficiency syndrome. *Journal of Applied Social Psychology, 17,* 216-230.

DiClemente, R.J., Zorn, J., & Temoshok, L. (1986). Adolescents and AIDS: A survey of knowledge, attitude and beliefs about AIDS in San Francisco. *American Journal of Public Health, 76,* 1443-1445.

Estrada, A.L., Dalgarn, R., deBoer, M., Fernandez, Stone, K., & Englander, S. (1989). *Knowledge, attitudes, beliefs and behaviors towards AIDS among Arizona Native Americans.* A paper presented at the American Public Health Association Conference in Chicago, October 23.

Evans, R.I., Roxelle, R.M., Mittlemark, M.B., Hansen, W.B., Bane, A., & Havis, J. (1978). Deterring the onset of smoking in children: Knowledge of immediate physiological effects and coping with peer pressure, media pressure, and parent modeling. *Journal of Applied Social Psychology, 8,* 126-135.

Flay, B.R. (1987). Mass media and smoking cessation: A critical review. *American Journal of Public Health, 77(11),* 153-160.

Flora, J.A., & Thoresen, C.E. (1989). Components of a comprehensive strategy for reducing the risk of AIDS in adolescents. In V.M. Mays, G.W. Albee, & S.F. Schneider (Eds.), *Primary prevention of AIDS: Psychological Approaches, Vol. XIII* (pp. 374-389). Newbury Park: Sage Publications.

Flora, J.A., & Thoresen, C.E. (1988). Reducing the risk of AIDS in adolescents. *American Psychologist, 43(11),* 965-970.

Freimuth, V., Edgar, T., & Hammong, S. (1987). College students awareness and interpretation of the AIDS risk. *Science, Technology, & Human Values, 12(3 & 4).*

Gilchrist, L.D., & Schinke, S.P. (1983). Coping with contraception: Cognitive and behavioral methods with adolescents. *Cognitive Therapy and Research, 7(5),* 379-388.

Gilchrist, L.D., Schinke, S.P., Trimble, J.E., & Cvetkovich, G.T. (1987). Skills enhancement to prevent substance abuse among American Indian adolescents. *The International Journal of Addictions, 22(9),* 869-879.

Glynn, T.J., Leukefeld, C.G., & Ludford, J.P. (Eds.)(1983). Preventing adolescent drug abuse: Intervention strategies. *NIDA Research Monograph 47.*

Goodman, E., & Cohall, A.T. (1989). Acquired immunodeficiency syndrome and adolescent minority population. *Pediatrics, 84(1),* 36-42.

Hayes, C.D. (Ed.). (1987). *Risking the future: Adolescent sexuality, pregnancy, and childbearing, Volume I.* Washington, D.C.: National Academy Press.

Hein, K. (1989). AIDS in adolescence: Exploring the challenge. *Journal of Adolescent Health Care, 10,* 10s-35s.

Hingson, R.W., Strunin, L., Berline, B.M., Heeren, T. (1990). Beliefs about AIDS, use of alcohol and drugs, and unprotected sex among Massachusetts adolescents. *American Journal of Public Health, 80(3),* 295-300.

Hofferth, S.L., & Hates, C.D. (Eds.). (1987). *Risking the future: Adolescent sexuality, pregnancy, and childbearing, Volume II.* Washington, D.C.: National Academy Press.

Janz, N.K., & Becker, M.H. (1984). The health belief model: A decade later. *Health Education Quarterly, 11,* 1-47.

Johnston, L.D., Bachman, J.G., & O'Malley, P.M. (1987). *Drug use among American high school students, college, and other young adults: National trends through 1986.* Rockville, MD: National Institute on Drug Abuse.

Kegeles, S.M., Adler, N.E., & Irwin, C.E. (1988). Sexually active adolescents and condoms: Changes over one year in knowledge, attitudes and use. *American Journal of Public Health, 78,* 460-461.

Kenney, A.M., Guardado, S., & Brown, L. (1989). Sex education and AIDS education in the schools: What states and large school districts are doing. *Family Planning Perspectives, 21(2)*, 56-64.

Kirby, D. (1984). *Sexuality education: An evaluation of programs and their effects*. Santa Cruz: Network Publications.

Lisken, L., Church, C.A., Piotrow, P.T., & Harris, J.A. (1989). AIDS education - A beginning. *Population Reports, 17(3)*, 1-32.

McGuire, W.J. (1964). Inducing resistance to persuasion. In L. Berkowitz (Ed.), *Advances in experimental social psychology* (Vol. 1, pp. 191-229). New York: Academic Press.

Melton, G.B. (1988). Adolescents and prevention of AIDS. *Professional Psychology: Research and Practice, 19(4)*, 403-408.

Miller, L. & Downey, A. (1987). *Knowledge and attitude change in adolescents following 1 hour of AIDS instruction*. Presented at the Third International Conference on AIDS, Washington, D.C. June 2.

National Institute on Drug Abuse (1986). *Prevention research: Deterring drug abuse among children and adolescents*. Research Monograph 63.

Penkey, J., Baldwin, J., Rolf, J., Platt, M., Perry, M., & Alexander, C. (1990). *Maryland Evaluation Project of the Red Cross HIV/AIDS Prevention Program for Youth*. Final Report.

Perloff, L.S. (1987). Social comparison and illusions of invulnerability to negative life events. In C.R. Snyder & C.E. Ford (Eds.), *Coping with negative life events* (pp. 217-242). New York: Plenum Press.

Platt, M., Baldwin, J., Rolf, J., Perry, M., Alexander, C., & Pankey, J. (1990). *Long term follow-up of student behavioral responses to a widely used HIV/AIDS prevention curriculum.* Abstract submitted to American Public Health Association Conference for September, 1990.

Platt, M., Rolf, J., Baldwin, J., Perry, M., Alexander, C., & Pankey, J. (1990). *Becoming sexually active: Transition predictors from an AIDS prevention study.* Post presented at the Society for Research on Adolescents, March, 1990.

Price, J.H., Desmond, S., & Kukulka, G. (1985). High school students' perceptions and misperceptions of AIDS. *Journal of School Health, 55,* 107-109.

Reuben, N., Hein, K., & Drucker, E. (1988, March). *Relationship of high-risk behaviors to AIDS knowledge in adolescent high school students.* Paper presented at Society for Adolescent Medicine Annual Research Meeting, New York.

Rolf, J., Alexander, C., Chandra, A., Baldwin, J., Jang, G., Armao, F., & Sorensen, M. (1989). *AIDS knowledge and vulnerabilities in Native vs. Non-Native American youth.* Presented at the American Public Health Association Conference in Chicago, October 23.

Rolf, J., Nanda, J., Baldwin, J., Chandra, A., & Thompson, L. (in press - 1990). Substance misuse and HIV/AIDS risks among delinquents: A prevention challenge. *The International Journal of Addiction, 25(3).*

Rudd, R.E., Kichen, J.M., & Joslin, I.D. (1980). *Student produced health education material: The photonovella. A how-to manual.* Easthampton, MA: Lifeways/Health Promotion Resource Center.

Schinke, S.P. (1984). Preventing teenage pregnancy. In M. Hersen, R.M. Eisler, & P.M. Miller (Eds.), *Progress in behavior modification* (pp. 32-64). San Francisco: Academic Press.

Shafer, M.A. (1988). High risk behavior during adolescence. In R.F. Schinazi & A.J. Nahmias (Eds.), *AIDS in children, adolescents, & heterosexual adults. An interdisciplinary approach to prevention* (pp. 323-324). New York: Elsevier.

Sonenstein, F.L., Pleck, J.H., Ku, L.C. (1989). Sexual activity, condom use and AIDS awareness among adolescent males. *Family Planning Perspectives, 21(4),* 152-158.

Sorenson, R.C. (1973). *Adolescent sexuality in contemporary America: Personal values and sexual behavior.* New York: Abrams.

Strunin, L., & Hingson, R. (1987). Acquired Immunodeficiency Syndrome and adolescents: Knowledge, beliefs, attitudes and behaviors. *Pediatrics, 79,* 825-828.

Telch, M.J., Killen, J.D., McAlister, A.L., Perry, C.L., & Maccoby, N. (1982). Long-term follow-up of a pilot project on smoking prevention with adolescents. *Journal of Behavioral Medicine, 5,* 1-8.

Tolsman, D.D. (1988). Activities of the Centers for Disease Control in AIDS education. *Journal of School Health, 58,* 133-136.

U.S. Congress, Office of Technology Assessment (1988). *How effective is AIDS education?* (Staff paper). Washington, D.C.: Government Printing Office.

Vermund, S.H., Hein, K., Gayle, H.D., Cary, J.M., Thomas, P.A., & Drucker, E. (1989). Acquired immunodeficiency syndrome among adolescents: Case surveillance profiles in New York City and the rest of the United States. *American Journal of Diseases of Children, 143, 1220-1225.*

Washington Post (1988, May 17). Adolescents: AIDS epidemic's next hot spot. Vulnerability of sexually active teenagers concerns public health officials.

Watkins, J.D. (1988). Responding to the HIV epidemic: A national strategy. *American Psychologist, 43(11),* 849-851.

Zabin, L.S., Kantner, J.F., & Zelnik, M. (1979). The risk of adolescent pregnancy in the first months of intercourse. *Family Planning Perspectives, 11(4),* 215-222.

Zelnik, M. (1983). Sexual activity among adolescents: Perspectives of a decade. In E.R. McAnaery (Ed.), *Premature adolescent pregnancy and parenthood.* New York: Grune & Stratton.

Zelnik, M., & Shah, S.K. (1983). First intercourse among young Americans. *Family Planning Perspectives, 15(2),* 64-70.

Table 1. Outcome and Process Objectives of the Harford County -
Red Cross HIV/AIDS Prevention Evaluation Project

A. Short-term Objectives

Proportions of students demonstrating Positive increases:

1. 80% in HIV/AIDS knowledge
2. 70% in self-efficacy beliefs with regard to health-promoting behaviors
3. 50% in communications with peers about AIDS
4. 50% in perception of personal HIV risk
5. 60% in motivation to learn more about HIV prevention
6. 70% in attitudinal dispositions towards prevention

B. Longer-term Objectives

Proportions of students retaining intervention gains at 1 year follow-up:

1. 50% regarding HIV/AIDS knowledge and preventive attitudes towards
   AIDS
2. 30% regarding implementation of AIDS relevant risk avoidance behaviors (e.g., delay
   of initiation of sexual intercourse, or if sexually active, consistent and proper
   use of condoms)

C. Process Objectives:

1. The Red Cross curriculum with the role play and photonovel innovative interventions
   are feasible and are accepted by youth.
2. The project anticipated necessary steps to innovating and implementing the HIV/AIDS
   prevention programs.
3. The research team can identify and help overcome barriers to implementation.

Table 2. Baseline Characteristics – Demographic variables
By School

	School 1	School 2	School 3	School 4	School 5
Mean Age (SD[1])					
1st Semester	14.32 (0.70) (n=97)	14.10 (0.54) (n=145)	14.26 (0.64) (n=87)	14.16 (0.40) (n=75)	– –
2nd Semester	14.51 (0.75) (n=96)	14.35 (0.62) (n=159)	14.44 (0.81) (n=108)	14.30 (0.54) (n=73)	14.48 (0.75) (n=135)
Gender					
1st Semester	55.7% Male (n=97)	56.6% Male (n=145)	47.1% Male (n=87)	50% Male (n=76)	– –
2nd Semester	50% Male (n=96)	49.4% Male (n=158)	55.6% Male (n=108)	50% Male (n=74)	54.8% Male (n=135)
Race					
1st Semester	82.5% White (n=97)	90.3% White (n=145)	80.2% White (n=86)	92.1% White (n=76)	– –
2nd Semester	83.3% White (n=96)	94.3% White (n=159)	82.4% White (n=108)	97.3% White (n=74)	54.5% White[2] (n=134)

[1] SD= Standard deviation

[2] 30.6% Black

Table 3. Categories of Variables and Types of Questions Included in the Surveys

1. Demographics

    - Age, Sex, Race, Grade Level of Subject
    - Where and with Whom Subject Lives
    - Parents' Occupation and Education

2. Background Characteristics

    - Family values
    - Religious Beliefs
    - Future Orientation

3. HIV/AIDS Knowledge

    - General knowledge scale
    - Casual contact misconceptions scale
    - See Table 6 for items

4. Attitudes and Beliefs about HIV/AIDS

    - Perceived Severity of HIV/AIDS (i.e., no current cure)
    - Perceived Barriers to Preventive Actions
    - Perceived Risk of Infection for self and others
    - Perceived Benefits of Prevention Actions (i.e., using condoms)
    - Worry/concern about AIDS
    - Personally know anyone with AIDS, AIDS virus, or an STD

5. Self-efficacy Beliefs regarding HIV/AIDS prevention skills

    - 3 scales: sexual pressure resistance, HIV/AIDS prevention communication, positive
      assertion for prevention
    - (See Table 7 for items)

6. Types of Changes in Knowledge, Attitudes or Behavior reported after Intervention Units

    - Learned more about risks, seriousness & consequences of teen pregnancy
    - Learned more about risks, seriousness & consequences of AIDS
    - Will wait to have sex or abstain
    - Will use condoms
    - Intend to change behavior in some other way
    - Communicated with peers about HIV/AIDS
    - Discussed HIV/AIDS with sex partner
    - Able to refuse pressure to have sex
    - Succeeded in changing behavior in some other way

7. Communication with Parents

    - Communication with parents about dating, drugs, sex, pregnancy, STD's, AIDS
    - Comfort in talking with parents about AIDS and Teen Pregnancy

8. Communication with Peers, Peer Contact and Peer Support

    - HIV/AIDS communications
    - Degree to which friends are confided in
    - Degree to which would feel comfortable talking to friends about sexual decisions
    - Number of close friends
    - Amount of free time spent with friends

9. General Negative Assertion Scale from Buhrmester et al. (1988)

    - Same-Sex Friend
    - Opposite-Sex Friend

Table 3. Categories of Variables and Types of Questions Included in the Surveys (cont'd)

10. **Peer Norms (Same Age at Same School) Regarding:**

   - Sexual behavior, including perceived number of peers who:
       are sexually active,
       using condoms during sex,
       feel comfortable discussing AIDS and Teen Pregnancy,
       have gotten pregnant or STDs
   - Cigarette, alcohol, and other drug use

11. **Peer Pressure to:**

   - Have sex, use protection during sex
   - Smoke, drink alcohol, or use other drugs

12. **Sexual Behavior**

   - Experience in holding hands, hugging and kissing, petting, heavy petting, sexual
     intercourse
   - Age of first intercourse
   - Number of sexual experiences in life
   - Number of different sex partners
   - Use of birth control at first and last intercourse
   - Birth control method at first and last intercourse
   - Use of STD protection at first and last intercourse
   - STD prevention method used at first and last intercourse
   - Intending to use condom at next intercourse
   - Had sex while tipsy or high

13. **Dating Behaviors**

   - Steady boyfriend/girlfriend; how long in relationship
   - Number of people dated in past year; age of dates

14. **Drug Use**

   - Ever tried tobacco, alcohol, marijuana, inhalants, stimulants, depressants, cocaine,
     PCP, narcotics, hallucinogens
   - Frequency of use of drugs in the past month: alcohol, cigarettes, marijuana,
     inhalants, cocaine, stimulants, depressants, narcotics, hallucinogens
   - Age started regularly smoking, drinking, using marijuana
   - Frequency of drinking alcohol before, during, or after school
   - Ever shared needles to inject drugs
   - Availability of alcohol at social gatherings

15. **Risk-taking Behavior**

   - 9 item scale (Alexander et al. in press)

16. **Affective Mood**

   - Kandel Depressive Mood Scale
   - Six items from Spielberger's Trait Anxiety Scale

17. **Process Related Items**

   - Feedback on Red Cross video and materials
   - Comparison of Red Cross workbook to other health education material
   - Feedback on Photonovel (e.g., reality of characters, storyline, how enjoyable it was
     to read)
   - Comparison of photonovel to other readings
   - Feedback on role playing (e.g., aspects of role playing liked most, least,
     suggestions would make to improve)

Table 4. Baseline Data on Sexual Activity

	1st Semester	2nd Semester
	%	%
Sexually active.	33.8	40.1
	(n=388)	(n=424)

Of those reporting sexual activity:

Number of Partners

1	35.5	40.4
2	18.6	15.7
3	16.2	15.1
>3	30.7	28.8
	(n=124)	(n=166)

Age Began Sexual Intercourse

<13	20.8	24.7
13	32.0	31.8
14	37.6	35.3
15	8.8	8.2
16	0.8	0
	(n=125)	(n=170)

Used condoms at last sexual intercourse

Yes	63.7	63.3

Table 5. Baseline Data on Sexual Activity By School

	School 1	School 2	School 3	School 4
Number sexually active				
1st Semester	35 (36%)	51 (35.2%)	23 (26.4%)	16 (21.1%)
2nd Semester[1]	51 (53.1%)	63 (39.6%)	43 (39.8%)	13 (17.6%)
Mean number of sexual partners (SD)				
1st Semester	2.79 (2.72)	4.40 (6.12)	4.27 (6.13)	4.33 (7.47)
2nd Semester[2]	3.39 (3.52)	3.39 (4.87)	6.17 (6.45)	1.85 (0.90)
Mean age of first intercourse (SD)				
1st Semester	13.03 (1.81)	12.86 (1.29)	13.43 (1.31)	13.75 (1.06)
2nd Semester	13.02 (1.22)	13.25 (1.40)	12.49 (2.00)	12.77 (1.88)
Used condom at last sexual intercourse				
1st Semester	57.1% (n=35)	70.5% (n=44)	63.2% (n=19)	68.8% (n=16)
2nd Semester	57.8% (n=45)	73.2% (n=56)	52.8% (n=36)	70.0% (n=10)

[1]significant school difference, X^2=23.65, 3 df, p<.001
[2]significant school difference, F (3,165) = 4.23, p<.01

Table 6. HIV/AIDS Knowledge Items and Mean Scale Scores at Baseline,
Immediate Posttest, & Subsequent Follow-up (Schools and
Semesters Combined)

HIV/AIDS Knowledge Items (superscript indicates scale membership)

True or False

[1] AIDS stands for Acquired Immune Deficiency Syndrome
[1] There is a blood test to detect infection with the AIDS virus
[1] A pregnant woman who has AIDS virus can give it to her unborn baby
[1] Vaginal intercourse is a way of getting AIDS
[1] Using a condom during sex can lower the risk of being infected with the AIDS virus
[1] At present, there is no cure for AIDS
[1] Only homosexuals get AIDS
[1] Teenagers have become infected with the AIDS virus

Among the different ways of getting infected with the AIDS virus, what are the chances if a
person does the following things? (Chances are relatively high or low)

[1]   Goes to school with a student who has AIDS
[1,2,3] Uses an infected person's belongings, like a comb or hair brush
[1,2]   Receives a blood transfusion with infected blood
[3]   Swims in a pool with someone who has the AIDS virus
[3]   Donates blood
[1]   Has unprotected sex (i.e., no condom) with a person infected with the AIDS virus
[3]   Is bitten by a mosquito which has also bitten someone who has the AIDS virus
[1,2]   Has sex with many different people
[3]   Eats in a restaurant where the cook has the AIDS virus
[1]   Shares needles (syringes) to inject a drug
[1,2]   Shakes hands or hugs someone who is infected with the virus
[1,2,3] Comes into contact with the saliva (spit) or tears of a person infected with the AIDS
         virus

| | | Mean Scores (Standard Deviation) | | |
HIV/AIDS Knowledge Scale Scores	Baseline	Immediate Posttest	2 Month Follow-up	6 Month Follow-up
16-item HIV/AIDS knowledge scale[1]	14.04 (2.21)	15.22 (1.55)*		
5-item HIV/AIDS knowledge scale[2]	4.07 (.96)	4.61 (.73)*	4.45 (1.02)*	4.45 (1.02)
HIV/AIDS Misconception scale[3]	3.39 (1.71)	5.14 (1.25)*	4.99 (1.43)*	

*Paired t-test comparisons between baseline to posttest and baseline to follow-up assessment
were significant at p<.001

Table 7. The Second Semester Self-efficacy Scales: Items,
Descriptive Statistics & Psychometric Properties
(Males & females combined)

Items	Item Range	Item x (SD)	Factor Reliability	Eigen-value
Factor 1 - Sexual Pressure Resistance Efficacy			α =.80	4.06
1) How sure can say no to sex with a boy/girl friend when pressured	0-100%[a]	60.8 (33.3)		
2) How sure can say no to sex with a new date when pressured	"	65.2 (31.7)		
3) How sure can resist pressure from peers to have sex	"	65.5 (28.8)		
Factor 2 - HIV/AIDS Prevention Communication Efficacy			α =.73	1.38
1) How sure can talk with boy/girl friend about AIDS & related topics	0-100%[a]	73.7 (24.7)		
2) How sure can talk with a parent about AIDS & related topics	"	58.4 (32.8)		
3) How sure can talk with friends about AIDS & related topics	"	73.2 (26.1)		
Factor 3 - Positive Assertion Efficacy			α =.73	1.00
1) How sure can insist on using condoms during intercourse	0-100%[a]	85.6 (21.1)		
2) How sure can consistently practice AIDS preventive behaviors	"	83.8 (19.8)		
3) How sure can ask new partner about previous sex/drug experiences	" .	68.7 (27.7)		
4) How sure can convince a friend to abstain from sex	"	68.8 (26.3)		

[a]Definitely Cannot do it		Probably Cannot		Maybe (50/50)			Probably Can		Definitely Can do it
0%	10%	20%	30%	40%	50%	60%	70%	80%	90%	100%

Table 8. Change in Self-Efficacy Scale Means by Gender: (Comparisons Between Baseline and Immediate Posttest and Between Baseline and Follow-up)

	N^a	Baseline	Immediate Posttest	Follow-up
Sexual Pressure Resistance Efficacy				
Males	192	52.82 (26.85)	54.90 (26.15)*	58.80 (27.94)*
Females	192	75.19 (21.67)	77.68 (21.24)*	82.54 (18.61)*
Both	384	64.00 (26.82)	66.29 (26.38)*	70.67 (26.52)*
HIV/AIDS Prevention Communication Efficacy				
Males	192	63.61 (23.35)	64.14 (22.45)*	68.20 (21.23)*
Females	192	73.31 (20.37)	76.22 (19.03)*	80.36 (17.15)*
Both	384	68.46 (22.42)	70.18 (21.65)*	74.28 (20.21)*
Positive Assertion Efficacy				
Males	192	72.84 (19.17)	69.28 (17.89)*	71.82 (16.73)*
Females	193	80.05 (16.25)	79.42 (17.18)*	82.91 (14.68)*
Both	385	76.46 (18.11)	74.36 (18.24)*	77.38 (16.67)*

Mean Scores (Standard Deviation)

^{a}N's represent students present at all time points.

Significance levels indicate paired t-test comparisons, baseline to immediate posttest and baseline to follow-up, respectively.

$\overset{*}{}$ p > .05
$\underset{.}{}$ p < .05

Table 9. Student-Parent Communication about HIV/AIDS and Related Topics
(Comparisons Between Baseline and Immediate Posttest
and Between Baseline and Follow-up)

Talked to parents about ...

Percent "Yes"

	Semester[a]	N[b]	Baseline	AIDS Posttest	Follow-up[c]
AIDS	1	302	46.5%	62.7%[*]	41.3%[*]
	2	385	33.8%	52.7%[*]	39.2%[*]
Teen Pregnancy	1	270	24.8%	41.5%[*]	28.1%[*]
	2	388	28.4%	33.5%[*]	40.2%[*]
STDs	1	300	29.7%	31.6%[*]	28.3%[*]
	2	386	15.5%	27.2%[*]	23.6%[*]
Sex	1	300	35.7%	48.7%[*]	
	2	404	35.9%	38.1%[*]	
Dating	1	302	57.6%	60.6%[*]	
	2	407	62.9%	52.6%[*]	
Drugs	1	302	55.6%	55.3%[*]	
	2	404	57.2%	51.5%[*]	

[a] 1st semester had Teen Pregnancy Unit before the AIDS Unit
[b] N's represent students present at all time points
[c] Follow-up for 1st semester = 6 months, 2nd semester = 2 months; only topics
assessed at follow-up were AIDS, Teen pregnancy and STD's.

Significance levels indicate McNemar comparisons within the same semester,
baseline to immediate posttest and baseline to follow-up, respectively.

[*] p > .05
[*] p < .05

Table 10. Percentages of Students at each Assessment Who
have Spoken to Peers about AIDS Prevention

Percent "Yes"

	Semester	Baseline	Immediate Posttest	Follow-up[a]
Have you talked with any person your age about how to prevent getting AIDS?	1	33.2	52.3[bc]	11.8[d]
	2	35.9	34.9	13.8[d]
Percent who reported talking to 4 or more peers	1	15.6[b]	21.4[e]	6.5[f]
	2	9.9	19.3[e]	6.0[f]

[a] Follow-up at 6 months 1st semester, 2 months 2nd semester
[b] Cross semester differences, Chi sq $\geq$ 6.22, 1 df, p<.01
[c] Within semester changes baseline to immediate posttest, McNemar X^2=34.3, p<.001
[d] Within semester changes baseline to follow-up, McNemar $X^2 \geq$36.9, p<.001
[e] Within semester changes baseline to immediate posttest (0-3 person vs. 4 or more
persons), McNemar $X^2 \geq$4.6, p<.05
[f] Within semester changes baseline to follow-up (0-3 persons vs. 4 or more),
McNemar $X^2 \geq$3.84, p<.05

Figure 1. Diagram of Quasi-Experimental Design

<u>1st Semester</u>

Schools	
1	TP-RC-O_1-----------------------PN-$O_{6\,mos.}$-------------------$O_{12\,mos.}$
2,3,4	O-TP-O_1-RC-O_1--------------------------$O_{6\,mos.}$-------------------$O_{12\,mos.}$

<u>2nd Semester</u>

Schools	
1	O-RC+RP-O_1-TP------PN-$O_{2\,mos.}$------------------$O_{8\,mos.}$
2	O-RC+RP-O_1-TP---------$O_{2\,mos.}$------------------$O_{8\,mos.}$
3,4	O-RC-O_1-TP---------$O_{2\,mos.}$------------------$O_{8\,mos.}$
5	RC-O_1-TP---------$O_{2\,mos.}$------------------$O_{8\,mos.}$

<u>Key</u>

O - Assessments; O_1 - immediate posttest, O_2, O_6, O_8, O_{12} - follow-ups at 2, 6, 8, & 12 months
RC - Red Cross AIDS Prevention Program for Youth (5 class periods)
RC+RP - RC (3 days) + Peer model video and role play (2 days)
TP - Teen Pregnancy Unit
PN - Photonovel

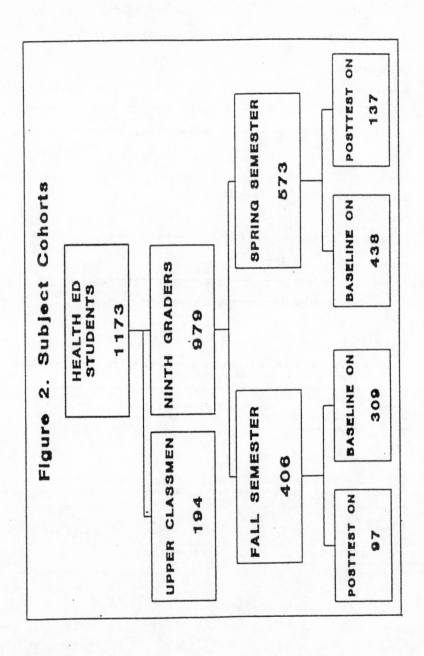

Figure 2. Subject Cohorts

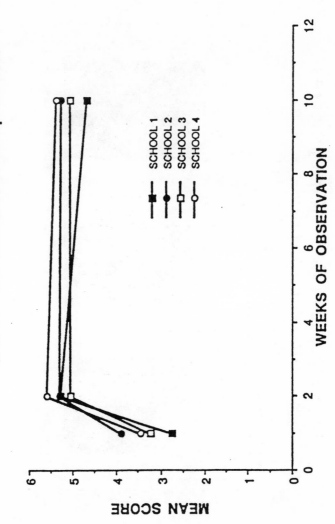

Figure 3. Mean Knowledge Scores (HIV/AIDS Misconceptions)

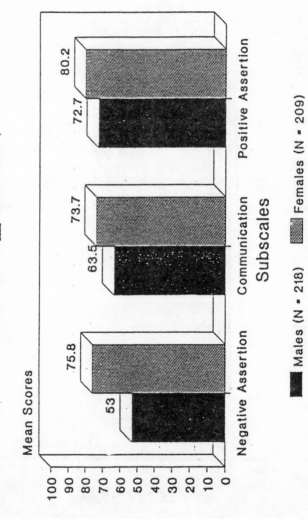

Figure 4. Mean Self-Efficacy Scores
(Baseline – 2nd Semester)

Neg. Assertion: F(1,426) = 96.92, p<.001
Communication: F(1,426) = 23.06, p<.001
Pos. Assertion: F(1,426) = 18.64, p<.001

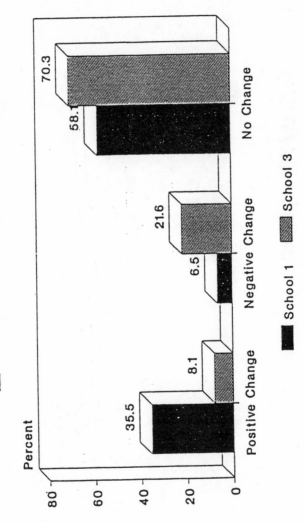

Figure 5. Self-Efficacy
Change in Resistance Skills For Females
2nd Semester (Baseline to Posttest)

Chi-Square = 9.17, 2 df, p=.01

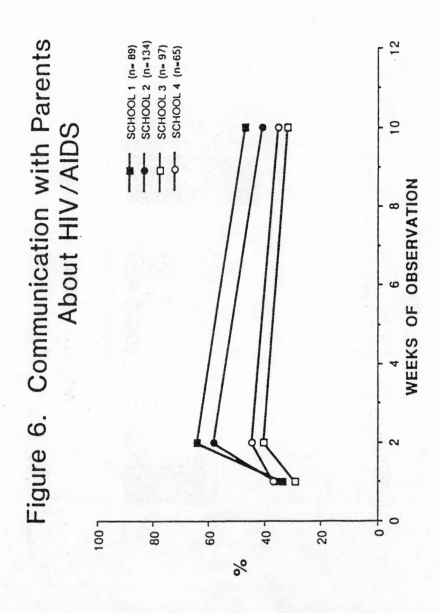

Figure 6. Communication with Parents About HIV/AIDS

2

AIDS PREVENTION: INTENTION OF HIGH SCHOOL STUDENTS TO USE CONDOMS

Joanne Otis

Gaston Godin

Jean Lambert

Using Fishbein and Ajzen's theory of reasoned action (1975) as conceptual framework, objectives for this study were: (1) to identify among students psychosocial factors likely to influence their intention to use condoms: (a) when the female partner is taking oral contraceptives, and (b) when the female partner is not taking the pill; (2) to establish whether or not these contexts directly affect intention; and (3) to evaluate whether or not the addition of variables external to the model could increase its predictive power. A sample of 1225 grade eleven students was asked to complete a questionnaire investigating the psychosocial variables. Regression of intention on all studied variables showed that personal normative beliefs, attitude, context, role belief, behavioral beliefs, and the interaction term between context and normative beliefs explained 64% of the total variation. Subjects had less intention of using condoms when the girl was taking the pill. Adding external variables to the theory of reasoned action increased its predictive value by 10%. Educational interventions in the school setting should address simultaneously the two roles of condoms: contraception and STD-AIDS prophylaxis. Condom use should be perceived by students as a socially desirable behavior, appropriate in the eyes of the social group they belong to, and highly in agreement with the moral values of those who adopt it.

Using Fishbein and Ajzen's theory of reasoned action (1975) as a conceptual framework, objectives for this study were the following:

1.   to identify among senior high school students, psychosocial factors influencing their intention to use a condom with a new partner, in two specific contexts: (a) where the female partner is taking oral contraceptives, and (b) where the female partner is not taking the pill;

2.   to establish whether or not these contexts directly affect intention;

3.   to evaluate whether or not the addition of external variables to the model increased its predictive power.

Results would be used initially to guide the planning of AIDS-STD prevention programs in the school setting and secondly, to establish basic parameters for evaluation of these programs. This research was also intended to demonstrate the usefulness of psychosocial models such as the theory of reasoned action for the planning process in health education.

Since 1981, AIDS has become epidemic and is now considered one of the most important public health issues in our society. People who are between 20 and 29 years of age account for approximately 20% of cases (Health and Welfare Canada, 1989). Given the long incubation period for the virus, a number of these cases have most probably been contracted during adolescence (Sunenblick, 1988). Even though the prevalence of AIDS among 15- to 19-year-olds is about 1%, it is estimated that the rate of seropositivity doubles every year within this age group (Brooks-Gunn, Boyer & Hein, 1988; Diclemente, Boyer & Mills, 1987). One of the reasons for this is that young people engage in unprotected sexual intercourse (Flick, 1986; Greer, 1981; Irwin & Millstein, 1986; O'Reilly & Aral, 1985; Zelnick & Kantner, 1980).

Condoms, when used appropriately, are a highly efficient barrier against HIV infection (CDC, 1988; Feldblum & Fortney,

1988; Stone, Grimes & Madger, 1986). Promotion of condom use seems to make sense among adolescents when compared to abstinence or other forms of sexual behavior modification (Rotheram-Borus & Koopman, 1989). However, prevalence of condom use remains low in spite of the few existing programs (Becker & Joseph, 1987; Solomon & DeJong, 1986).

According to recent studies, regular condom use varies from 0 to 31% among adolescents (Desjardins, Langlois & Lemoyne, 1986; Hingson, Strunin, Berlin, Heeren, 1990; Keleges, Adler & Irwin, 1988; Michaud & Hausser, 1989). Also, contraception and prophylaxis do not seem very compatible in this age group. Less than 15% of adolescents report having used simultaneously a condom and another contraceptive device (Riphagen, 1989; Valdiserri, Arena, Proctor & Bonati, 1989). Furthermore, for females, the rate of condom use decreases as they grow older, when they are taking the pill (Chapman & Hodgson, 1988; White & Johnson, 1988). It thus becomes imperative to identify and understand better which factors are likely to influence the decision-making process towards adoption of the use of condoms among young people (Becker, 1988; Kann, Nelson, Jones & Kolbe, 1989). In this regard, there is a need to differentiate between: (a) condoms as a protective measure against AIDS and other STD; and (b) condoms as a contraceptive method.

Up to now, numerous descriptive studies have tried to identify reasons for use or non-use of condoms as a contraceptive device (Flick, 1986; Galavotti & Lowick, 1989; Morrison, 1985; Solomon & DeJong, 1986). Fewer efforts have been directed at condom use as an STD prophylactic measure (Chapman & Hodgson, 1988; Strader & Beaman, 1989; Valdiserri, Arena, Proctor & Bonati, 1989). Some theoretical studies have been designed to identify the predictors of condom use among adolescents (Eisen, Zellman & McAlister, 1985; Katatsky, 1977; Morrison, 1985) and in this context, the theory of reasoned action seemed to stand out from others (Ewald & Roberts, 1985; Fisher, 1984; Jaccard & Davidson, 1972, 1975; Lavoie, 1989; McCarty, 1981; Pagel & Davidson, 1984; Traeen, Rise & Kraft, 1989). However, none of these studies tried to identify among the same population the determinants of condom use according to its double role: contraception and disease prevention. The present study was designed to fill this gap.

THEORETICAL FRAMEWORK

According to Fishbein and Ajzen (1975), intention (I), to perform a given behavior is a function of attitude towards this behavior, (Aact), and of the subjective norm governing this situation, (SN). Relative contribution of these two components may be determined using multiple regression techniques, these contributions being indicated by the standardized regression coefficient (W_1, W_2). Such weights may vary according to the behavior under study, the specific context, or respondent's characteristics. The regression equation is formulated as:

$$I = (Aact) \ W_1 + (SN) \ W_2.$$

Attitude (Aact), is itself determined by behavioral beliefs (perceived outcome: advantages and disadvantages) regarding adoption of the behavior. For each belief (b_i), the individual estimates the probability of the outcome being manifest and makes a subjective evaluation (e_i), of this outcome. This indirect measure of attitude is obtained by summation of the strength of each behavioral belief (b_i), weighted by its subjective evaluation (e_i). It is algebraically described as:

$$Aact = \sum_{i=1}^{n} b_i \times e_i.$$

Subjective norm (SN), corresponds to normative beliefs, that is, to perceived approval or disapproval from significant others (NB_j), towards this behavior, and to motivation to comply with their opinion (MC_j). Indirect measure of subjective norm is represented by the following equation:

$$SN = \sum_{j=1}^{m} NB_j \times MC_j.$$

Fishbein and Ajzen (1975) underlined the importance, in this theory, of taking into account the level of correspondence between measures of intention and other constructs of the model. This correspondence is established around four criteria: action, target, time, and context. Furthermore, the effect of external variables such as age, gender, personality, etc. should be mediated through the diverse elements of the model.

Given the health problem linked to the behavioral intention under study, an original aspect of this research consisted in establishing the relationship between the context ("with the pill" and "without the pill") and intention to use condoms. Context was considered to be an independent variable, a potential predictor of intention. Many researchers in the field of social psychology recognized the theoretical importance of context (Furnhamm & Argyle, 1981; Magnusson, 1981). For example, Kahle and Beathy have demonstrated that task situation was not a variable exogenous to the model, but rather a direct predictor of intention.

Furthermore, in order to increase the predictive value of the theory of reasoned action, six additional variables were considered. Choice was based on numerous studies demonstrating their importance when trying to predict intention. The first two concepts were taken from Ajzen's theory of planned behavior (1985). In its revision of the theory of reasoned action, Ajzen (1985) incorporated perception of behavioral control (PBC) as a new concept for the prediction of intention. The resulting regression equation is:

$$I = (Aact) \, W_1 + (SN) \, W_2 + (PBC) \, W_3.$$

Ajzen and Timko (1986, P262) defined the new concept this way: "Perceived behavioral control is similar to Bandura's (1977, 1982) self-efficacy construct." However, "perceived behavioral control was assumed to reflect external factors (e.g., availability or time or money, cooperation of other people, etc.) as well as internal factors (ability, skill, information, etc.)". "Self-efficacy" or "perceived behavioral control" have been found to be predictors of intention in many studies (Ajzen & Madden, 1986; Godin & Lepage, 1988; McCaul, O'Neil & Glasgow, 1988; Schifter & Ajzen, 1985), namely for intention to use a contraceptive or prophylactic method (Gilchrist & Schinke, 1983; Lavoie, 1989). Ajzen (1985) also proposed another way to measure perception of behavioral control. It consists of an evaluation of the prevailing environmental conditions that facilitate or hinder the performance of this behavior. In this regard, condom use could be influenced by barriers such as cost, embarrassment to buy, lack of ability to put on a condom, and by the adolescents' perception of "being in control" in this type of situation.

Two other variables were taken from Triandis's model (1977): "personal normative belief" (PNB), and "role belief" (RB). Personal normative belief corresponds to the moral obligation felt by the individual towards adopting a behavior. This variable increased the predictive value of the theory of reasoned action in many studies (Brindberg, 1979; Rausch, Lee & White, 1988; Valois, Desharnais & Godin, 1988; Zuckerman & Reiss, 1978), namely in prediction of intention to use a contraceptive method (Pagel & Davidson, 1984). Role belief was chosen as an alternative to the social norm concept of Fishbein and Ajzen (1975) (SN), which was found in recent studies as inappropriately defined (Lutz, 1976; Miniard & Cohen, 1981; Valois, Desharnais & Godin, 1988).

Past behavior was the fifth added variable. Its importance in predicting intention was widely demonstrated (Bentler & Speckart, 1979; Budd, North & Spencer, 1984; Godin & Shephard, 1986; Godin, Valois, Shephard & Desharnais, 1987). Moreover, Ewald and Roberts (1985) confirmed the predictive power of this variable for intention to use condoms among adolescents. Perception of health risk was the last predictor considered. According to Rosenstock (1974), this variable predicts behavior, and this has been confirmed in diverse studies concerned with use of contraceptive methods among adolescents (Condelli, 1986; Lowe & Radius, 1987; Nathanson & Becker, 1983).

Research hypothesis for this study was that these variables are all potential predictors of intention. It seemed important to identify, among these, the psychosocial factors most strongly linked with the young people's decision-making process towards condom use with a new partner, and this, according to two different contexts, "with the pill" and "without the pill."

METHODS

Sampling Procedure

The study population was drawn from male and female senior high school students, French- and English-speaking, attending 17 public or private schools, situated on Montreal's South Shore (total: 4702 students). Of the 17 schools eligible for the study, 14 accepted to participate (total: 4302 students). In order to include every school, they represented strata. A stratified one-stage cluster sampling with proportional allocation was used, classes being clusters. Sample size determination was based on the multiple regression analysis; with $\alpha = 0.01$, $B = 0.05$ and a possibility of 10 independent variables, a sample size of approximately 555 students by context was sufficient to detect a R^2 of as low as 0.05 (Cohen, 1988). Of the 1289 randomly selected subjects who filled out the questionnaire, 64 were dropped, due to missing data, leaving 1225 questionnaires (95%) for statistical analysis. No significant differences between respondents and non-respondents were observed.

Questionnaire

The final questionnaire was developed from a preliminary study conducted among a group of 181 students bearing similar characteristics to the study population. In this preliminary study, subjects were administered an open-ended questionnaire. Following the methodology proposed by Ajzen and Fishbein (1980), they were asked to enumerate perceived advantages and disadvantages, perceived barriers relating to the use of condoms with a new partner, and to list the people who according to them would agree or disagree with this behavior. By randomization, half of the students were asked to answer questions in the context of the female partner taking the pill, and the other half in the context of the girl not taking the pill. Based on this information, and using the most frequently mentioned elements, the main study questionnaire was elaborated. Four slightly different versions were prepared, specific for male or female respondents, and the two contexts; "with" or "without" the pill. The resulting questionnaires were validated among nurses, teachers, and other subgroups of students for clarity and simplicity. In order to establish the psychometric value of the instrument, 343 students were administered these final versions. Internal consistency of each construct under study, calculated by Cronbach's alpha, varied from 0.66 to 0.79. Sixty-nine of these students were also submitted to a test-retest evaluation within a three week interval. Intra-class correlation coefficients calculated for each construct from the test-retest, varied from 0.60 to 0.92.

Data Collection

Considering these results as satisfactory, the selected students were informed of the study objectives during a short meeting, a month before the actual testing they were given the questionnaire in the spring of 1989 during regular classes. Within each classroom, the versions were randomly distributed according to both contexts. Directives were read to each group at the time of testing. Students were reminded that the questionnaire would be anonymous, that they were free to participate or not, and that the questionnaire was intended for everyone, sexually active or not. Answering time was about 40 minutes.

Study Variables

For reasons of simplicity, the examples presented below refer to the formulation for boys.

All variables measured according to the "taking the pill" or "not taking the pill" contexts included the following hypothetical situation: "If during the next two months, I engaged in sexual intercourse with a new partner who takes the pill." (or does not take the pill). Sexual intercourse was defined as "penetration of the penis."

Intention (I). The score for intention was obtained by the summation of two items. For the first item, the student was asked to what degree he "would be determined to use a condom" and for the second, to what degree he "would intend to use a condom."

The first scale varied from *not at all* (1) to *extremely* (7); the second went from *definitely not* (-3) to *definitely* (+3). Theoretically, score for intention could vary from (-2) to (+10).

Attitude towards the act (Aact). Subjects reported their attitude towards the behavior on eight semantic differential scales, ranging from (-3) to (+3). The bipolar adjectives were: disagreeable-agreeable; useless-useful; irresponsible-responsible; repulsive-attractive; unpleasant-pleasant; immoral-moral; thoughtless-thoughtful; and cumbersome-convenient. Each of the eight scales appeared following the statement: ". . . actual use of condoms would be . . . for me." Global score for attitude ranged from (-24) to (+24). Internal consistency was tested by using Cronbach's alpha coefficient; an appropriate value of 0.79 was found.

Behavioral beliefs $(\Sigma \ b_i \ x \ e_i)$. Advantages and disadvantages identified from the preliminary study were the following: the use of a condom would: "protect me from contracting STD," "make me feel safer," "prevent my new sexual partner from becoming pregnant," "interrupt the progress of intercourse," "decrease my sexual pleasure," "be annoying," "make me feel that sexual intercourse was less natural," "make me worry that the condom would break," and "introduce a feeling of distrust between my partner and me." The strength of each belief (b_i) was measured on a scale from (-3) *extremely unlikely* to (+3) *extremely likely* for advantages and from (+3) to (-3) for disadvantages. Evaluation of consequences (e_i) offered a seven level unipolar scale, ranging from *neither good, nor bad* (0) to the *best of all* (6) for positive consequences or to *worse than anything* (6) for negative consequences. Global score was obtained by summation of each probability, (b_i), weighted by its evaluation, (e_i). Consequently, behavioral beliefs varied from (-162) to (+162). Internal consistency for this construct reached 0.67.

Subjective norm (SN). Subjective norm was obtained by asking students to what degree people who are important to them "would approve or disapprove of their using condoms" in this context. A bipolar scale ranging from *totally disapprove* (-3) to *totally approve* (+3) was used.

Normative beliefs (Σ NB$_j$ x MC$_j$). Significant people mentioned during the preliminary study were: "my parents," "my friends," "my sexual partner," "doctors." For each category of significant persons, subjects had to indicate if they would "agree or disagree with the fact that I use a condom." Each item, (NB$_j$), varied from *completely disagree*, (-3), to *completely agree*, (+3). In order to measure motivation to comply, (MC$_j$), the following question was asked: "relating to the use of condoms, I would be . . . inclined to act according to the opinion of. . . ." Their answers could go from *not at all*, (1), to *definitely*, (7). Summation of the strength of each normative belief, (NB$_j$), weighted by motivation to comply, (MC$_j$), constituted the global score for this construct. It could vary from (-84) to (+84). Cronbach alpha was 0.65.

Perceived behavioral control (PBC). As measured by summation of two items, global score for this construct went from (-2) to (+10). Subjects were asked: (1) "using condoms or not would . . . *definitely not*, (-3), to *definitely*, (+3), be up to me," (2) "the fact that we use a condom or not would . . . *not at all*, (1), to *definitely*, (7), . . . depend on me."

Perceived barriers. For each barrier listed in the preliminary study, the student had to identify to what degree it would be easy or difficult for him: "to buy condoms himself," "to assume the cost of condoms," "to get condoms when he wants, in different places," "to convince his new sexual partner to use condoms," "to put on a condom," "to always have condoms on hand at the time of intercourse." Each item was assessed on a scale ranging from *extremely difficult*, (+3), to *extremely easy*, (-3). Summation of all items could go from (-18) to (+18), accounting for the global score of the perceived barriers. This construct obtained a Cronbach alpha coefficient of 0.77.

Personal normative belief (PNB). Moral obligation was measured by the following question: ". . . my own principles make me believe that I should . . . *definitely not*, (-3), to *definitely*, (+3), . . . use condoms."

Role belief (RB). A single bipolar item was chosen to measure this concept. Students were asked ". . . is it appropriate or inappropriate for boys of your age (Secondary 5) to use condoms with a new partner "if the girl takes the pill" or "if the girl does not take the pill." The scale ranged from *extremely inappropriate*, (-3), to *extremely appropriate*, (+3).

Perception of risk. Perception of risk was measured by three items. The first item related to risk of pregnancy; the second related to the risk of contracting AIDS; the third related to the risk of contracting an STD other than AIDS. Each item was put on a scale from *nil*, (1), to *extremely high*, (7). After a principal component analysis, it was decided not to group these three elements. Only the items relating to risk of STD and AIDS were included, giving a score from (+2) to (+14). Risk of pregnancy was treated independently.

Habit (H). Among the sexually active, data was collected relating to the protective method used during the first intercourse (condom, pill, etc.). Subjects were also asked what proportion of their sexual intercourses were protected by the pill or condoms since the first intercourse. (Four categories were constituted: *none; a minority of; most of; all of.*)

Context (C). Context was coded for purpose of analysis in the following fashion: (0) in the context where the girl is not taking the pill, and (1) in the context where the girl is taking the pill.

Other external variables. Diverse socio-demographic variables such as age, ethnic group, etc. . . . were gathered. Among sexually active subjects, other data relating to their sexual behaviors were also sought.

Statistical Analysis

Multiple stepwise regression analyses were used to identify predictors of intention. Predictors were considered for inclusion, if all the following criteria were met: (1) an empirical significance level less than 0.01 ($p<0.01$); (2) a standardized partial regression coefficient of at least 0.10; (3) an increment in the adjusted R^2 of at least 0.75%. Interactions between context and other variables were considered also for inclusion. Aptness of final models were studied through analysis of residuals.

RESULTS

The final sample was composed of 1225 students, females representing 54.7% of the group. Mean age for respondents was 17.11 ± 0.61 years ($X \pm$ S.D.). At the time of the study, the majority (74.9%) of the students were living with both parents. 38.4% of the boys and 48.7% of the girls reported having a steady girl or boyfriend. Furthermore, 61.4% of the boys and 57.6% of the girls mentioned they had at least one sexual intercourse with penetration. Results concerning this sub-group of sexually active students are presented in Table 1. (747 students were sexually active; due to missing data, 658 questionnaires [88%] were used for analysis purposes.) Among these sexually active young people, a higher proportion of boys declared they had six or more different sexual partners (14.2% for the boys; 8.2% for the girls). However, 22.7% of the boys and 16.3% of the girls reported that all their sexual intercourse was protected by a condom.

Descriptive results for study variables are presented in Table 2. It can be observed that among our respondents intention to use condoms with a new partner was relatively high, particularly in the context where the girl is not taking oral contraceptives. In this context, intention reached a mean value of 8.50 ± 1.82 on a scale from (-2) to (+10), compared to a mean score of 6.74 ± 2.90 when the girl is taking the pill. This difference between contexts was observed for the majority of the constructs under study.

The correlation matrix indicated a moderate association between attitude (Aact), and behavioral beliefs (Σ be), (r=0.52), and between subjective norm (SN), and normative beliefs (Σ NBMC), (r=0.34). However, though statistically significant, the correlation between perception of behavioral control (PBC) and perceived barriers was quite weak (r=-0.11).

Results for stepwise multiple regression will present the predictive value of: (1) the theory of reasoned action (Fishbein and Ajzen, 1975); (2) the theory of planned behavior (Ajzen, 1985); (3) a model including Triandis's variables (1977) and external variables of interest.

1. *The Theory of Reasoned Action*

    Multiple regression for all constructs from the theory of reasoned action and their respective interactions with the variable context (pill versus no pill) showed that six predictors of intention explained 55% of the total variation (adjusted R^2). Context was the best predictor with a standardized partial regression coefficient of -0.51. Attitude (Aact) was the second best predictor reaching a partial regression weight of 0.28. The additional significant predictors were the interaction term between the context and attitude (C x Aact), subjective norm (SN), the interaction term between context and normative beliefs (C x Σ NBMC), and behavioral beliefs (Σ be).

2. *The Theory of Planned Behavior*

    The consideration of the variables from the theory of planned behavior (perceived behavioral control [PBC] and perceived barriers) and their interaction term with context, showed a regression model where seven predictors of intention yielded an adjusted R^2 of 0.56. The six predictors taken from the theory of reasoned action remained within the model, in the same order and with similar partial regression weights. However, perception of behavioral control was added.

3. *Triandis's Variables Added to Model*

    In the final model, Triandis's variables (personal normative beliefs [PNB], role belief [RB]), and variables relating to health risk were added. Their respective interactions with context were considered. Six variables explained 65% of the total variation. These were in order of importance: (1) personal normative beliefs (PNB); (2) attitude (Aact); (3) context; (4) interaction term between context and normative beliefs (C x Σ NBMC); (5) behavioral beliefs (Σ be); and (6) role belief (RB).

At the end, respondents' sociodemographic characteristics and sexual activity status were considered for inclusion in the final model. None of these variables reached significance. Furthermore, after gathering supplementary data among sexually active students about their sexual practices and preventive behaviors (use of the pill, of condoms, number of partners, etc.), the same regression steps were performed among this group. A model similar to the one shown in Table 6 was obtained, with the same six predictors explaining 64% of the total variation. Past behavior did not reach a significant weight for the prediction of intention.

DISCUSSION

Students in our sample reported preventive and sexual behaviors similar to previous observations cited in the literature for this age group (Flick, 1986; Hingson, Strunin, Berlin & Heeren, 1990; King, Beazley, Warren, Hankins, Robertson & Radford, 1988; Leslie-Warwitt & Meheus, 1989; Strunin & Hingson, 1987; Zelnik & Kantner, 1980). Moreover, intention to use condoms with a new partner was at a higher level in the context where the girl does not take the pill. Intention remained rather positive, but to a lesser degree, in the context where the female partner uses the pill. The "new partner" situation is probably responsible for this relatively strong desire to use condoms either way.

In agreement with the works of Miller and Ginter (1979) and Kalhe and Beatty (1989), the present results positively support the importance of context as a predictive variable for intention. As maintained by Fishbein & Ajzen (1975, 1976), in different contexts, a quite different predictive model for each context can be obtained. In this regard, in the context where the girl is taking the pill, a direct effect of the adolescents' normative beliefs on their intention was noted. Thus, when protected from the risk of pregnancy, adolescents feel direct social pressures concerning the use of condoms. These pressures seem to originate from the influence of significant people, such as friends, sexual partners, parents, and physicians.

Considering the theory of reasoned action by itself, the results are in agreement with numerous other studies relating to adolescents' intention to use condoms (Ewald & Roberts, 1985; Fisher, 1984; Jaccard & Davidson, 1972; Lavoie, 1989; Traëen, Rise & Kraft, 1989). As in the present study, most of these works showed that attitude was the best predictor.

Furthermore, according to the theory of planned behavior, the addition of the variables proposed by Ajzen (1985) contributed very weakly to the prediction of intention, increasing the total explained variation by only 1%. Perception of behavioral control was the sole additional variable to reach a sufficient weight. Similar results were obtained by Lavoie (1989). He observed an increment of 2% in the predictive value of this model. As suggested by Ajzen and Madden (1986), there could be a gap between one's perception of behavioral control and actual control over the decision. Taking this hypothesis into account, perception of control could be a direct predictor of behavior, not of intention. Nevertheless, for the prediction of intention to use condoms with a new partner, the theory of reasoned action and the theory of planned behavior seemed to reach the same power of prediction.

The predictive value of the model was increased with the addition of personal normative belief. This was in agreement with the findings of Pagel and Davidson (1984), who reported that personal normative belief was a better predictor of intention to use a contraceptive method than were behavioral beliefs and normative beliefs. According to Budd and Spencer (1984, 1985) and Kashima and Kashima (1988), personal normative belief reflects a greater internalization of social influences. Thus, given the magnitude of the AIDS phenomenon over the recent years, the contribution of personal normative belief suggests that a certain moral obligation, a kind of social responsibility, prevails among students. Furthermore, during adolescence, people share role beliefs with their peers. This was supported by the addition of role belief into the model. Thus, making reference to one's social group influences the decision-making process toward the use of condoms, in both contexts.

Surprisingly, contrary to observations by Ewald and Roberts (1985) and Lavoie (1989), the prediction of intention to use condoms was not influenced by past behavior. Thus, the use of condoms in the past does not increase the chances that someone will form a positive intention towards their use. In this regard, it is possible to see past behavior to predict directly future behavior. This needs to be further analyzed in prospective studies. Perception of health risk did not influence intention to use condoms. This suggests that among people of this age category, it is unlikely that the fear of a health problem will play on the decision-making process regarding the intention to use condoms. Finally, the influence from socio-demographic variables (age, gender, ethnic origin, family structure, etc.) was mediated through the constructs of the model. This supported Fishbein and Ajzen's (1975) postulate and was in accordance with a number of other works (Jaccard & Davidson, 1975; Timko, 1987).

Implications for Intervention

Personal factors have a major influence in the adolescents' decision-making process towards the use of condoms. These factors take the form of a moral obligation that is felt or not felt towards use of condoms with a new partner and of a more or less positive attitude towards this behavior. At the attitudinal level, both cognitive and affective dimensions are important. We feel that educational strategies should promote the following messages: condom use with a new partner is a very desirable behavior; the individual who behaves this way shows a high sense of social responsibilities; furthermore, this behavior is totally in accordance with his or her personal principles and moral values. This should be done taking both contexts simultaneously. In order to develop a more positive attitude among young people, messages should reinforce the advantages perceived with condom use: its double protective value and the feeling of safety it can bring. On the other hand, whether rational or emotional, disadvantages must be played down, even contradicted (e.g., condoms reduce pleasure versus condoms prolong duration of intercourse and thus can increase pleasure).

Social factors are also linked to decision-making. It is of the utmost importance to take into account membership in a social group. It must be established clearly that condom use with a new partner is an appropriate behavior for a 17-year-old boy or girl.

Students should be comfortable in affirming that this behavior is essential if they are to be "a class act." Furthermore, when the matter is approached according to the context where the girl is already taking the pill, special attention should be paid to normative beliefs: probable agreement from friends or from the eventual sexual partner should be stated, explained, and proven. In this regard, educational efforts in the school setting should address the pregnancy and STD/AIDS problems simultaneously. Students' normative beliefs in both contexts should be confronted. Students have to understand why they feel these different social pressures and they should develop the necessary skills to cope with these influences.

However, in the perspective of AIDS and STD prevention, one prerequisite should be met in order to make the results of the present study readily usable: it must be made absolutely clear among adolescents that a new, regular boy or girlfriend is technically a new sexual partner. Educational programs must avoid limiting the debate to what might otherwise be perceived as applying only to casual sex. In the present study, this was insisted upon prior to the subjects' answering the questionnaire.

This study permitted identification of determinants of young peoples' decision towards the use of condoms with a new partner and one of its major contributions was to show the importance of the contraceptive and prophylactic contexts in regard to this decision. Whether intention accurately predicts behavior in our sample remains to be assessed; the prospective chapter of this work will enable us to test this hypothesis in the near future.

REFERENCES

Ajzen, I. (1985). From intentions to actions: A theory of planned behavior. In J. Kuhl & J. Beckman (Eds). *Action-control: From cognition to behavior.* Heidelberg, Springer, 11-39.

Ajzen, I. & Fishbein, M. (1980). *Understanding attitudes and predicting social behavior.* Englewood Cliffs, NJ: Prentice-Hall.

Ajzen, I. & Madden, T.J. (1986). Prediction of goal-directed behavior: Attitudes, intentions, and perceived behavioral control. *Journal of Experimental Social Psychology, 22,* 453-474.

Ajzen, I. & Timko, C. (1986). Correspondence between health attitudes and behavior. *Basic and Applied Social Psychology, 7(4),* 259-276.

Bandura, A. (1977). Self-efficacy: Toward a unifying theory of behavioral change. *Psychological Review, 84,* 191-215.

Bandura, A. (1982). Self-efficacy mechanism in human agency. *American Psychologist, 37(2),* 122-147.

Becker, M.H. (1988). AIDS and behavior change. *Public Health Reviews, 16,* 1-11.

Becker, M.H. & Joseph, J.G. (1987). AIDS and behavioral change to reduce risk: A review. *American Journal of Public Health, 78(4),* 394-410.

Bentler, P.M. & Speckart, G. (1979). Models of attitude behavior relations. *Psychological Review, 86(5),* 452-464.

Brindberg, D. (1979). An examination of the determinants on intention and behavior: A comparison of two models. *Journal of Applied Social Psychology, 9(6),* 560-575.

Brooks-Gunn, J., Boyer, C.B., & Hein, K. (1988). Preventing HIV infection and AIDS in children and adolescents: Behavioral research and intervention strategies. *American Psychologist, 43,* 958-964.

Budd, R.J., North, D. & Spencer, C.P. (1984). Understanding seat-belt use: A test of Bentler and Speckart's extension of the theory of reasoned action. *European Journal of Social Psychology, 14(1)*, 69-78.

Budd, R.J. & Spencer, C.P. (1984). Predicting undergraduate's intentions to drink. *Journal of Studies on Alcohol, 45(2)*, 179-182.

Budd, R.J. & Spencer, C.P. (1985). Exploring the role of personal normative beliefs in the theory of reasoned action: The problem of discriminating between alternative path models. *European Journal of Social Psychology, 15*, 299-313.

CDC (1988). Condoms for prevention of sexually transmitted diseases. *Public Health Reviews, 16*, 13-19.

Chapman, S. & Hodgson, J. (1988). Shower in raincoats: Attitudinal barriers to condom use in high-risk heterosexuals. *Community Health Studies, 12(1)*, 97-105.

Cohen, J. (1988). *Statistical power analysis for the behavioral sciences*. Lawrence Erlbaum Associates. Hillsdale, NJ.

Condelli, L. (1986). Social and attitudinal determinants of contraceptive choice: Using the health belief model. *Journal of Sex Research, 22(4)*, 478-491.

Desjardins, M.F., Langlois, S. & Lemoyne, Y. (1986). Enquête épidémiologique sur la sexualité d'adolescents fréquentant un cegep. *L'Union Médicale du Canada, 115*, 668-671.

DiClemente, R.J., Boyer, C.B., & Mills, S.J. (1987). Prevention of AIDS among adolescents: Strategies for the development of comprehensive risk-reduction health education programs. *Health Education Research, 2(3)*, 287-291.

Eisen, M., Zellman, G.L. & McAlister, A. (1985). A health belief model approach to adolescents' fertility control: Some pilot program findings. *Health Education Quarterly, 12(2),* 185-210.

Ewald, B.M. & Roberts, C.S. (1985). Contraceptive behavior in college-age males related to Fishbein model. *Advances in Nursing Science, 7(3),* 63-69.

Feldblum, P.J. & Fortney, J.A. (1988). Condoms, spermicides, and the transmission of human immunodeficiency virus: A review of literature. *American Journal of Public Health, 78(1),* 52-54.

Fishbein, M. & Ajzen, I. (1975). *Belief, attitude, intention and behavior: An introduction to theory and research,* Reading, Massachusetts: Addison-Wesley.

Fishbein, M. & Ajzen, I. (1976). Misconceptions about the Fishbein model: Reflections on a study by Songer-Nocks. *Journal of Experimental Social Psychology, 12,* 579-584.

Fisher, W.T. (1984). Predicting contraceptive behavior among university men: The role of emotions and behavioral intentions. *Journal of Applied Social Psychology, 14(2),* 104-123.

Flick, L.M. (1986). Paths to adolescent parenthood: Implications for prevention. *Public Health Reports, 101,* 132-147.

Furnham, A., & Argyle, M. (Eds.) (1981). *The psychology of social situation: Selected readings.* Oxford: Pergamon.

Galavotti, C. & Lovick, S.R. (1989). School-based clinic use and other factors affecting adolescent contraceptive behavior. *Journal of Adolescent Health Care, 10,* 506-512.

Gilchrist, L.D. & Schinke, S.P. (1983). Coping with contraception: Cognitive and behavioral methods with adolescents. *Cognitive Therapy and Research, 7(5),* 379-388.

Godin, G. & Lepage, L. (1988). Understanding the intentions of pregnant nullipara to not smoke cigarettes after childbirth. *Journal of Drug Education, 18(2),* 115-124.

Godin, G. & Shephard, R. (1986). Psychosocial factors influencing intentions to exercise of young students from grade 7 to 9. *Research Quarterly for Exercise and Sport, 57(1),* 41-52.

Godin, G., Valois, P., Shephard, R. & Desharnais, R. (1987). Prediction of leisure time exercise behavior: A path analysis (LISREL V) model. *Journal of Behavioral Medicine, 10(2),* 145-158.

Greer, J.G. (1981). Psychosexual issues in adolescent contraception. *Public Health Reviews, 10(1),* 27-47.

Health and Welfare Canada (1989). AIDS Surveillance in Canada. *Canada Diseases Weekly Report, 15-52,* 259-260.

Hingson, R.W., Strunin, L., Berlin, B.M., & Heeren, T. (1990). Beliefs about AIDS, use of alcohol and drugs, and unprotected sex among Massachusetts adolescents. *American Journal of Public Health, 80(3),* 295-299.

Irwin, C.E. & Millstein, S.G. (1986). Biopsychosocial correlates of risk-taking behaviors during adolescence. *Journal of Adolescent Health Care, 7,* 82S-96S.

Jaccard, J.J. & Davidson, A.R. (1972). Toward an understanding of family planning behaviors: An initial investigation. *Journal of Applied Social Psychology, 2(3),* 228-325.

Jaccard, J.J. & Davidson, A.R. (1975). A comparison of two models of social behavior: Results of a survey sample. *Sociometry, 38(4)*, 497-517.

Kahle, L.R. & Beatty, S.E. (1987). The task situation and habit in the attitude-behavior relationship: A social adaptation view. *Journal of Social Behavior and Personality, 2(2)*, 219-232.

Kann, L., Nelson, G.D., Jones, J.T., & Kolbe, L.G. (1981). Establishing a system of complementary school-based surveys to annually assess HIV-related knowledge, beliefs, and behaviors among adolescents. *Journal of School Health, 59(2)*, 55-58.

Kashima, Y. & Kashima, E.S. (1988). Individual differences in the predictions of behavioral intentions. *The Journal of Social Psychology, 128(6)*, 711-720.

Katatsky, M. (1977). The health belief model as a conceptual framework for explaining contraceptive compliance. *Health Education Monographs, 5(3)*, 232-243.

Keleges, S.M., Adler, N.E., & Irwin, C.E. (1988). Sexually active adolescents and condoms: Changes over one year in knowledge, attitudes and use. *American Journal of Public Health, 78(4)*, 460-461.

King, A.J.C., Beazley, R.P., Warren, W.K., Hankins, C.A., Robertson, A.S., & Radford, J.L. (1988). *Etude sur les jeunes Canadiens face au SIDA.*

Lavoie, M. (1989). *La théorie de l'action raisonnée: application à l'usage du condom comme moyen de prévention des MTS.* Unpublished master's theses, Department of Social and Preventive Medicine, Université de Montréal.

Leslie-Warwit, M. & Meheus, A. (1989). Sexually transmitted disease in young people: The importance of health education. *Sexually Transmitted Diseases, 16(1),* 15-20.

Lowe, C.S., & Radius, S.M. (1987). Young adult's contraceptive practices: An investigation of influences. *Adolescence, 22(86),* 291-304.

Lutz, R.J. (1976). Conceptual and operational issues in the extended Fishbein model. *Advances in Consumer Research, 3,* 469-476.

Magnusson, D. (Ed.)(1981). *Toward a psychology of situations: An interactional perspective.* Hillsdale, NJ: Lawrence Erlbaum.

Manstead, A.S.R., Plevin, C.E., & Smart, J.L. (1984). Predicting mothers' choice of infant feeding method. *British Journal of Social Psychology, 23,* 223-231.

McCarty, D. (1981). Changing contraceptive usage intentions: A test of the Fishbein model of intention. *Journal of Applied Social Psychology, 11(3),* 192-211.

McCaul, K.D., O'Neil, H.K., & Glasgow, R.E. (1988). Predicting the performance of dental hygiene behaviors: An examination of the Fishbein and Ajzen model and self-efficacy expectations. *Journal of Applied Social Psychology, 18(2),* 114-128.

Michaud, P.A., & Hausser, D. (1989). La sexualité des adolescents à l'heure du SIDA. *Revue Médicale de la Suisse Romande, 109,* 319-326.

Miller, K.E., & Ginter, J.L. (1979). An investigation of situational variation in brand choice behavior and attitude. *Journal of Marketing Research, 16,* 111-123.

Miniard, P.N. & Cohen, J.B. (1981). An examination of the Fishbein-Ajzen behavioral-intentions model's concepts and measures. *Journal of Experimental Social Psychology, 17,* 309-339.

Morrison, D.M. (1985). Adolescent contraceptive behavior: A review. *Psychological Bulletin, 98(3),* 538-568.

Nathanson, C.A. & Becker, M.H. (1983). Contraceptive behavior among unmarried young women: A theoretical framework for research. *Population and Environment, 6(1),* 39-59.

O'Reilly, K.R., & Aral, S.O. (1985). Adolescence and sexual behavior. *Journal of Adolescent Health Care, 6,* 262-270.

Pagel, M.D., & Davidson, A.R. (1984). A comparison of three socio-psychological models of attitude and behavioral plan: Prediction of contraceptive behavior. *Journal of Personality and Social Psychology, 47(5),* 517-533.

Rausch, J.C., Lee, J., & White, R. (1988). Cigarette use among Alabama student nurses: An application of the theory of reasoned action. *Advances in Health Education, 1,* 203-217.

Riphagen, F.E. (1989). Contraception and AIDS prevention. *Contraception, 39(5),* 577.

Rosenstock, I. (1974). The health belief model and preventive health behavior. *Health Education Monographs, 2(4),* 354-386.

Rotheram-Borus, M.J., & Koopman, C. (1989). Safer sex and adolescence. In R. Herner, A. Peterson, J. Brooks-Bunn (Eds.), *Encyclopedia of Adolescence,* (in press). New York: Garland Press.

Schifter, D.E., & Ajzen, I. (1985). Intention, perceived control, and weight loss: An application of the theory of planned behavior. *Journal of Personality and Social Psychology, 49(3)*, 843-851.

Solomon, M.Z., & DeJong, W. (1986). Recent sexually transmitted disease prevention efforts and their implications for AIDS health education. *Health Education Research, 13(4)*, 301-316.

Stone, K.M., Grimes, D.A., & Madger, L.S. (1986). Primary prevention of sexually transmitted diseases. *Journal of the American Medical Association, 225(13)*, 1763-1766.

Strader, M.K., & Beaman, M.L. (1989). College students' knowledge about AIDS and attitudes toward condom use. *Public Health Nursing, 6(2)*, 62-66.

Strunin, L., & Hingson, R. (1987). Acquired immuno-deficiency syndrome and adolescents: Knowledge, beliefs, attitudes, and behaviors. *Pediatrics, 79(5)*, 825-828.

Sunenblick, M.B. (1988). The AIDS epidemic: Sexual behaviors of adolescents. *Smith College Studies in Social Work, 59(1)*, 21-37.

Timko, C. (1987). Seeking medical care for a breast cancer symptom: Determinants of intentions to engage in prompt or delay behavior. *Health Psychology, 6(4)*, 305-328.

Traëen, B., Rise, J., & Kraft, P. (1989). Condom behavior in 17, 18, and 19 year-old norwegians. *Proceedings of the V International Conference on AIDS*. Montreal, Quebec, Canada, p. 737.

Triandis, H.C. (1977). *Interpersonal behavior*. Brooks/Cole, Monterey, CA.

Valdiserri, R.O., Arena, V.C., Proctor, D., & Bonati, F.A. (1989). The relationship between women's attitudes about condoms and their use: Implications for condom promotion programs. *American Journal of Public Health, 79(4)*, 499-501.

Valois, P., Desharnais, R., & Godin, G. (1988). A comparison of the Fishbein and Ajzen and the Triandis attitudinal models for the prediction of exercise intention and behavior. *Journal of Behavioral Medicine, 11*, 459-472.

White, H.R. & Johnson, V. (1988). Risk taking as a predictor of adolescent sexual activity and use of contraception. *Journal of Adolescent Research, 3(3-4)*, 317-331.

Zelnik, M., & Kantner, J.F. (1980). Sexual activity, contraceptive rise and pregnancy among metropolitan-area teenagers: 1971-1979. *Family Planning Perspectives, 12*, 230-237.

Zuckerman, M., & Reiss, H.T. (1978).   Comparison of three models for predicint altruistic behavior. *Journal of Personality and Social Psychology, 36(5)*, 498-510.

TABLE 1
Descriptive analysis of the sample of sexually active students (n=658)

Variables	Boys (n=308)	Girls (n=350)	p
Sexually active	61.4%	57.6%	NS
Current affective relationship			
none	47.4%	31.1%	
one year or less	38.3%	40.3%	**
more than one year	14.3%	28.6%	
Age at the time of the first intercourse	15.08 years	14.96 years	NS
Use of a contraceptive method at the first intercourse			
none	23.1%	31.1%	
pill	20.1%	16.3%	NS
condom	56.8%	52.6%	
Number of sexual intercourse			
five or less	32.1%	21.7%	*
more than six	67.9%	78.3%	
Number of different sexual partners			
only one	31.2%	39.4%	
between two and five	54.6%	52.4%	**
six or more	14.2%	8.2%	
Sexual intercourses protected by the use of condoms			
none	14.3%	24.6%	
a few	38.0%	46.5%	**
most of	25.0%	12.6%	
all of	22.7%	16.3%	
Sexual intercourses protected by the use of the pill			
none	26.9%	36.0%	
a few	35.1%	28.6%	NS
most of	18.5%	19.7%	
all of	19.5%	15.7%	
Belief of having contracted an S.T.D.	6.8%	26.9%	**
Previously treated for S.T.D.	2.3%	7.7%	*

** p < 0.0001
* p < 0.005

TABLE 2
Descriptive statistics for the studied constructs (n=1225)

Variables	With the pill $\bar{x} \pm$ s.d.	Without the pill $\bar{x} \pm$ s.d.	p
Intention (I)	6.74 ± 2.90	8.50 ± 1.82	**
Attitude-towards-the act (Aact)	6.67 ± 6.51	8.62 ± 5.91	**
Subjective norm (SN)	1.89 ± 1.26	2.28 ± 1.16	**
Behavioral beliefs (ΣBE)	28.44 ± 29.21	31.22 ± 27.36	NS
Normative beliefs (ΣNBMC)	25.52 ± 17.67	29.87 ± 16.74	**
Perceived behavioral control (PBC)	6.04 ± 2.95	6.52 ± 2.81	*
Perceived barriers	-5.75 ± 6.47	-7.08 ± 6.57	**
Personal normative belief (PNB)	1.75 ± 1.43	2.57 ± 0.90	**
Role belief (RB)	2.07 ± 1.32	2.58 ± 1.29	**
Risk of pregnancy	2.45 ± 1.14	5.01 ± 1.83	**
Risk of AIDS - S.T.D.	9.03 ± 3.31	8.03 ± 3.49	**

** $p < 0.0001$
* $p < 0.01$

TABLE 3

Correlation matrix of studied constructs. (n=1225)

Variables	1	2	3	4	5	6	7	8	9	10	11
1. Intention (I)	-										
2. Attitude (Aact)	0.62*	-									
3. Subjective norm (SN)	0.42*	0.27*	-								
4. Behavioral beliefs (ΣBE)	0.45*	0.52*	0.19*	-							
5. Normative beliefs (ΣNBMC)	0.35*	0.30*	0.34*	0.24*	-						
6. Perceived behavioral control (PBC)	0.29*	0.17*	0.14*	0.09	0.12*	-					
7. Perceived barriers	-0.14*	-0.12*	-0.08	-0.15*	-0.09	-0.11*	-				
8. Personal normative belief (PNB)	0.71*	0.50*	0.44*	0.32*	0.32*	0.25*	-0.11*	-			
9. Role belief (RB)	0.42*	0.29*	0.28*	0.23*	0.25*	0.09	-0.12*	0.35*	-		
10. Risk of pregnancy	0.29*	0.16*	0.12*	0.05	0.12*	0.08	0.02	0.28*	0.13*	-	
11. Risk of AIDS - S.T.D.	0.11*	0.12*	0.09	0.08	0.01	0.04	0.11*	0.10*	0.02	0.28*	-
12. Context (C)	-0.34*	-0.15*	-0.16*	-0.05	-0.13*	-0.08	0.10*	-0.33*	-0.19*	-0.64*	0.15*

* $p < 0.0001$

TABLE 4
Stepwise multiple regression analysis of intention to use a condom with
a new partner (n=1225)

Theory of reasoned action - Fishben & Ajzen (1975). (TRA)

Variables	Unstandardized partial regression coefficient b ± SE(b)	Standardized partial regression coefficient B ± SE(B)	p
1. TRA			
Attitude (Aact)	0.11 ± 0.010	0.28 ± 0.030	*
Subjective norm (SN)	0.42 ± 0.040	0.20 ± 0.020	*
Behavioral beliefs (Σ BE)	0.01 ± 0.002	0.15 ± 0.020	*
2. Others			
Interaction between Context and Attitude (C x Aact)	0.10 ± 0.020	0.23 ± 0.040	*
Interaction between Context and normative beliefs (C x Σ NBMC)	0.02 ± 0.004	0.17 ± 0.030	*
Context[1] (C)	-2.64 ± 0.180	-0.51 ± 0.040	*
Constant	6.13 ± 0.150		*

Overall R^2 adj. = 0.55; f = 249.80; p < 0.0001

* p < 0.0001

1. Context was coded: (0) without the pill, (1) with the pill.

TABLE 5
Stepwise multiple regression analysis Intention to use a condom with
a new partner (n=1225)

Theory of planned behavior - Ajzen (1985). (TPB)

Variables	Unstandardized partial regression coefficient $b \pm SE(b)$	Standardized partial regression coefficient $B \pm SE(B)$	p
1. TRA			
Attitude (Aact)	0.11 ± 0.010	0.26 ± 0.030	*
Subjective norm (SN)	0.39 ± 0.040	0.19 ± 0.020	*
Behavioral beliefs (ΣBE)	0.01 ± 0.002	0.15 ± 0.020	*
2. TPB			
Perceived behavioral control (PBC)	0.10 ± 0.020	0.12 ± 0.020	*
3. Others			
Interaction between Context and Attitude (C x Aact)	0.10 ± 0.020	0.22 ± 0.040	*
Interaction between Context and normative beliefs (C x Σ NBMC)	0.02 ± 0.004	0.16 ± 0.030	*
Context[1] (C)	-2.57 ± 0.180	-0.50 ± 0.030	*
Constant	5.54 ± 0.180		*

Overall R^2 adj. = 0.56; f = 225.67; p < 0.0001

* p < 0.0001

1. Context was coded: (0) without the pill, (1) with the pill.

TABLE 6
Stepwise multiple regression analysis of intention to use a condom with
a new partner (n=1225)

Theory of planned behavior and external variables from Triandis (1977).

Variables	Unstandardized partial regression coefficient b ± SE(b)	Standardized partial regression coefficient B ± SE(B)	p
1. TRA			
Attitude (Aact)	0.10 ± 0.010	0.25 ± 0.020	*
Behavioral beliefs (ΣBE)	0.01 ± 0.001	0.12 ± 0.020	*
2. Variables from Triandis			
Personal normative belief (PNB)	0.88 ± 0.040	0.43 ± 0.020	*
Role belief (RB)	0.23 ± 0.040	0.12 ± 0.020	*
3. Others			
Interaction between Context and normative beliefs (C x Σ NBMC)	0.02 ± 0.004	0.14 ± 0.030	*
Context[1] (C)	-1.20 ± 0.140	-0.23 ± 0.030	*
Constant	4.38 ± 0.130		*

Overall R^2 adj. = 0.65; f = 377.84; p < 0.0001

* p < 0.0001

1. Context was coded: (0) without the pill, (1) with the pill.

3

THE DEVELOPMENT AND EVALUATION OF A COMPREHENSIVE KNOWLEDGE SURVEY REGARDING AIDS

Mark J. Kittleson
John S. Venglarcik

The purpose of this study was to evaluate a comprehensive knowledge survey on AIDS and HIV transmission. A review of literature reveals an overabundance of attitudinal-based research studies, with limited efforts made at ascertaining current knowledge levels of HIV transmission. This study employed over 500 subjects to develop and evaluate a comprehensive survey to address basic modes of HIV transmission that was developed with the cooperation of university health care professionals, public health officials, and a hospital epidemiologist. Reliability was determined by various techniques, with subjects including over 300 health care workers. An item-by-item analysis revealed reliability ranging from .80 to 1.0. The results indicate that this instrument is a credible instrument that can be used as a source of pre- or post evaluation.

Acquired Immunodeficiency Syndrome (AIDS) has emerged as the number one public health concern of the 1980s and appears to continue as such as we enter into the 1990s. Presently, education appears to be a viable tool to reduce the spread of the disease and to quiet unwarranted fears. However, when one develops an educational program it is imperative that the needs of the participants be met (Pollock, 1987; Mathews, Mullen & Mast, 1979).

As the health care profession prepares to deal with the increasing numbers of AIDS patients and HIV infected individuals, up-to-date information regarding the disease and its transmission, as well as discussing the attitudinal aspects of caring for people infected with HIV needs to take place. Unfortunately, many of these programs are developed without identifying what health care workers need to know (Allen & Curran, 1988). Wertz et al. (1987) state that many health care workers, including physicians, have many misunderstandings regarding AIDS and HIV transmission, that can be altered with proper in-service. Identifying the needs can be accomplished in a variety of ways, but it is essential that such attempts are made prior to providing educational programs.

This study is an attempt to evaluate a broad-based, comprehensive, and simple questionnaire that addresses myths and misconceptions associated with AIDS and HIV transmission. It is hoped that such an instrument can be used to assist in the planning of effective and efficient AIDS education programs.

Figure 1 identifies the 56 item questionnaire. It is divided into two parts. Part 1 consists of 38 various modes of transmission. The questionnaire lists modes in one of four categories: casual contact, blood, sexual, and transplacentally. A review of literature has shown that the only modes of transmission that have been documented are through sexual contact (CDC, 1987a), blood (Friedland & Klein, 1987), and transplacentally, including breast milk (Ziegler et al., 1985). Many of the modes identified in the survey have a "theoretical" possibility (e.g., CPR on mannikin infected with HIV), but there has been no documented evidence of any transmission occurring that way (CDC, 1987a; Savitter et al., 1985).

Part 2 consists of 18 statements that the respondent must address as either "true" or "false." These questions tend to be clustered in the same four categories as the modes of transmission in Part 1.

VALIDITY

When one reviews validity, various dimensions of validity must be examined. Face validity does give the impression that this survey is valid.   Unfortunately, face validity is not always scientifically sound (Adams & Schvaneveldt, 1985).   To address the concerns of the content validity, all current findings regarding the transmission of HIV were investigated.   It is also important to point out that this survey is requesting relatively simple answers in a very complex area of health and medicine.

Transmission of HIV has been well-documented by the Centers for Disease Control.   In Figure 1, Part 1, the only documented modes of transmission identified by the literature and endorsed by the Centers for Disease Control are Question 5 - receiving blood from infected person (Curran et al., 1984), Question 6 - infected mother to fetus (Lapointe et al., 1985), Question 16 - mother's breast milk to infant (Lepage et al., 1987), Questions 21-23 - various forms of oral sex (Spitzer & Weiner, 1989; CDC, 1988; Mayer & Degruttola, 1987; Monzon & Capellan, 1987; Marmor et al., 1986), Questions 24-27 - various forms of intercourse (Laurian, Peynet & Verroust, 1989; Padian et al., 1987; CDC, 1987b; Friedland & Klein, 1987; Kingsley et al., 1987), and Question 36 - infected patient to medical worker in professional contact (CDC, 1987b; McCray et al., 1986).

Of the 18 statements in Part 2, Questions 39, 40, 42, 43, 47, 50, and 54 are all true.   The remaining questions are either totally false, or have components in the statements that are false, thus making the entire statement false.

PROCEDURES

The questionnaire was originally designed in the summer of 1987, and has had several revisions since then.   The original development of the instrument came after discussion and review of common misconceptions regarding the transmission of the HIV that were most often asked to their authors in their many discussions and presentations to professionals and lay groups.   A review of literature revealed the lack of a simple, as well as comprehensive evaluation to measure the knowledge level of how the HIV is transmitted.   With this in mind, the authors developed an instrument that would be relatively simple to complete, and provides a wide range of "theoretical" and "factual" modes of transmission to test the knowledge level of the respondent.

After development, the original instrument was given to 120 college students enrolled in a general health education class in a midwestern university. The purpose of this initial distribution was to discover the readability and clarity of the instrument. Besides answering the questions, the subjects were asked to mark on the actual instrument anything that was not clearly understood. An additional 120 college students enrolled in a general health class were also given the opportunity to complete this revised instrument, and they too were asked to identify those statements that were still unclear. After the second revision, 30 medical residents at two local teaching hospitals, and 30 university professors were also given the opportunity to complete and comment on the instrument. The instrument appearing in Figure 1 is the final result of those revisions.

Careful attention was made to allow the survey to be properly understood by various health care workers. Readability was determined by the use of the SMOG instrument. Assessment indicated that this instrument was written for an eighth-grade reading level. Although this level may be too high for a large proportion of the general public, it was felt by the researchers that health care workers would be able to read at that grade level. A careful analysis of the instrument indicates that certain polysyllabic words could be replaced with simpler terms. For example, when sex is replaced for intercourse, the reading level drops to 6th grade.

RESULTS

Reliability was tested in two methods. In the fall of 1988, 240 subjects enrolled in six college general health education classes (mean age was 24) were given a test-retest of the instrument 14 days apart. The class did not discuss AIDS or any other sexually transmitted diseases within these seven days. Fortunately during this two-week time period, little national attention by the media was given to AIDS. The reliability as determined by the Pearson Product Coefficiency was .891.

The second aspect of the reliability assessment was an item by item analysis of each statement. Item by item analysis was ascertained by using the same 240 subjects' scores. Reliability was determined by the use of the Phi Coefficiency. This technique was used because it is the preferred measurement when both variables are dichotomies (Hinkle, Wiersma & Jurs, 1979). Of the 56 items, 54 had correlations above +.80. From these results, it appears that the test is reliable from administration to administration. Two of the statements had correlations below .80 and were discarded. Figure 2 shows the items with acceptable correlations.

The final aspect of determining reliability was to measure the internal consistency of this survey among health care workers. Although the prior subjects (college students) were helpful in the early stages of instrument development, the authors acknowledge that there are vast differences in maturity, understanding, and knowledge between college students and health care workers. In an attempt to determine whether this instrument was reliable among health care workers, 325 physicians, nurses, and laboratory technicians completed the questionnaire, and their results were assessed to determine the internal consistency of the test. Each of the items in the two parts were randomly selected and placed in one of two parts.

Because of the difficulties associated with doing a test-retest reliability study among these subjects, the Spearman-Brown formula was used to assist in the determination of the reliability coefficiency. The reliability coefficiency for this, when adjusted by the Spearman-Brown Formula, was .912. To check further for internal consistency, Cronbach's Alpha revealed a score of .81, further indicating a reliable and consistent instrument (Cronbach, 1951).

DISCUSSION

The purpose of this survey was to assist in the development of a simple, yet comprehensive instrument that identifies theoretical (yet unsubstantiated) and documented modes of HIV transmission. Unfortunately, many of the already existing instruments do not specifically address the various modes identified in this survey. This questionnaire can elicit responses regarding specific misinformation as well as correct information. Based upon the two test-retest reviews, this instrument appears to be highly reliable.

The ramifications of possessing a reliable and valid instrument on a subject such as AIDS can be an enormous asset when developing and evaluating AIDS education programs. This is especially relevant to the health care profession, or those individuals involved extensively in AIDS education or counseling. In many instances, in-service directors have limited time to provide AIDS education. It is hoped that, by knowing areas of misunderstanding, such programs can focus directly on those areas.

REFERENCES

Adams, G.R., Schvaneveldt, J.D. (1985). *Understanding research methods.* White Plains, NY: Longman Inc.

Allen, J.R., Curran, J.W. (1988). Prevention of AIDS and HIV infection: Needs and priorities for epidemiologic research. *American Journal of Public Health, 78,* 381-386.

Centers for Disease Control (1988). Guidelines for effective school health education to prevent the spread of AIDS. *MMWR,* 1.

Centers for Disease Control (1987a). Human immunodeficiency virus infection in the United States: A review of current knowledge. *MMWR, 36* (suppl No. S-6), 36.

Centers for Disease Control (1987b). Update: Human immunodeficiency virus infection in health-care workers exposed to blood of infected patients. *MMWR, 36,* 285.

Cronbach, L. (1951). Coefficient alpha and the internal structure of tests. *Psychometriks, 16,* 297-334.

Curran, J.W., Lawrence, D.N., Jaffe, H., et al. (1984). Acquired immunodeficiency syndrome (AIDS) associated with transfusion. *New England Journal of Medicine, 310,* 69.

Friedland, G.H., Klein, R.S. (1987). Transmission of the human immunodeficiency virus. *New England Journal of Medicine, 317,* 1125.

Hinkle, D.E., Wiersma, W., Jurs, S.G. (1979). *Applied statistics for the behavioral sciences.* Boston: Houghton Mifflin Co.

Kingsley, L.A., Kaslow, R., Rinaldo, C.R., et al. (1987). Risk factors for seroconversion to human immunodeficiency virus among male homosexuals. *Lancet, 1,* 345.

Lapointe, N., Miahaud, J., Pekovic, D., et al. (1985). Transplacental transmission of HTLV-III virus. *New England Journal of Medicine, 312,* 1325.

Laurian, Y., Peynet, J., Verroust, F. (1989). HIV infection in sexual partners of HIV-seropositive patients with hemophilia. *New England Journal of Medicine, 320,* 183.

Lepage, P., Van de Perre, P., Carael, M., et al. (1987). Postnatal transmission of HIV from mother to child. *Lancet, 2,* 400.

Marmor, M., Weiss, L.R., Lyden, M., et al. (1986). Possible female-to-female transmission of human immunodeficiency virus. *Annals of Internal Medicine, 105,* 969.

Mathews, B.P., Mullen, P.D., Mast, E.M. (1979). Hospital-based health education: For patients, staff, and the community. *Health Values, 3(1),* 32-36.

Mayer, K.H., & Degruttola, V. (1987). Human immunodeficiency virus and oral intercourse. *Annals of Internal Medicine, 107,* 428.

McCray, E., et al. (1986). Occupational risk of the acquired immunodeficiency syndrome among health care workers. *New England Journal of Medicine, 313,* 1127.

Monzon, O.T., & Capellan, J.M.B. (1987). Female-to-female transmission of HIV. *Lancet, 2,* 40.

Padian, N., Malrquis, L., Francis, D.P., et al. (1987). Male-to-female transmission of human immunodeficiency virus. *JAMA, 258,* 788.

Pollock, M. (1987). *Planning and implementing health education in schools.* Palo Alto, CA: Mayfield Publishing Company.

Saviteer, S.S., White, G.C., Cohen, M.S., & Jason, J. (1985). HTLV-III exposure during cardiopulmonary resuscitation. *New England Journal of Medicine, 313,* 1606-1607.

Spitzer, P.G. & Weiner, N.J. (1989). Transmission of HIV infection from a woman to a man by oral sex. *New England Journal of Medicine, 320,* 251.

Wertz, D.C., Sorenson, J.R., Liebling, L., et al. (1987). Knowledge and attitudes of AIDS health care providers before and after education programs. *Public Health Reports, 102,* 248-254.

Ziegler, J.B., Cooper, D.A, Johnson, R.O., et al. (1985). Postnatal transmission of AIDS-associated retrovirus from mother to infant. *Lancet, 1,* 896.

FIGURE 1

AIDS QUESTIONNAIRE

Which of the following methods have been documented by the literature, and supported by the Centers of Disease Control, to spread Human Immunodeficiency Virus-HIV, (aka the AIDS virus), the causative agent of AIDS? Mark A if it has been shown to spread the disease; Mark B if it has not been shown.

1. Hugging an HIV infected person.
2. Having an infected HIV person bite and break the skin.
3. Sharing of cigarettes, cigars, or pipes with an HIV infected person.
4. Uninfected person donating blood.
5. Receiving blood from an HIV infected person.
6. HIV infected mother to fetus.
7. HIV infected father to fetus.
8. Mosquitoes to person.
9. Lip kissing with an HIV infected person.
10. Tongue or "wet" kissing with an HIV infected person.
11. Sharing of eating utensils with an HIV infected person.
12. Sharing of toilet facilities with an HIV infected person.
13. Sharing of razors with an HIV infected person.
14. Sharing of toothbrushes with an HIV infected person.
15. Sharing of beds, linen, pillows with an HIV infected person.
16. HIV infected mother's breast milk to infant.
17. Having tears of a person with HIV touch you.
18. Being sneezed upon by an HIV infected person.
19. Being coughed upon by an HIV infected person.
20. Being breathed upon by an HIV infected person.
21. Mouth of uninfected person to penis contact with an HIV infected person.
22. Mouth of uninfected person to vulva/vagina contact with an HIV infected person.
23. Mouth of uninfected person to anus contact with an HIV infected person.
24. Anal intercourse with an HIV infected person.
25. HIV infected male to male intercourse.
26. HIV infected male to female intercourse.
27. HIV infected female to male intercourse.
28. HIV infected female to female sexual intimacies.
29. Male to animal intercourse.
30. Animal to male intercourse.
31. Female to animal intercourse.
32. Animal to female intercourse.
33. CPR instruction on manikins infected with HIV.

34. CPR on actual humans infected with HIV.
35. Being "spitted" upon by an HIV infected person.
36. HIV infected patient to medical worker from a needlestick.
37. Patient receiving injections from medical workers.
38. Swimming in a pool with a person infected with HIV.

The following statements are either true or false. Mark A if true, mark B if false.

39. A good significant way to reduce your chances of "catching" the AIDS virus is for both partners to remain faithful to each other and not use I.V. drugs.
40. The more sexual partners a person has, the greater the risk of "catching" the AIDS virus.
41. A positive HIV antibody test means you have AIDS.
42. A positive HIV antibody test means you have been exposed to the virus.
43. HIV can be transmitted even if the person lacks symptoms.
44. Most babies born with the AIDS virus develop natural immunities, thus they can live a normal life.
45. Less than 1% of pregnant women with HIV transmit the disease to the fetus.
46. Many HIV transmissions have occurred among children in the school setting.
47. The contraction of the AIDS virus can be prevented or reduced significantly if a person abstains from sexual intercourse.
48. Most HIV infected individuals have become infected by using I.V. drugs.
49. Vaginal sex is more likely to spread the AIDS virus than anal sex.
50. The contraction of the AIDS virus can be prevented or reduced significantly by using a condom.
51. There have been a few reported cases of blood donors becoming infected with HIV while donating their blood.
52. The contraction of the AIDS virus can be prevented or reduced significantly by having the male withdraw his penis just before ejaculation.
53. AIDS can be cured by large doses of antibiotics.
54. If one does not engage in certain "high risk" behaviors, there is almost no chance of contracting the AIDS virus.
55. The AIDS virus can remain infective in dried blood for several hours out of the body.
56. Nobody under 18 years of age has died of AIDS.

FIGURE 2

ITEM BY ITEM ANALYSIS

Which of the following methods have been documented by the literature, and supported by the Centers of Disease Control, to spread Human Immunodeficiency Virus-HIV, (aka the AIDS virus), the causative agent of AIDS? Mark A if it has been shown to spread the disease; Mark B if it has not been shown.

1. Hugging an HIV infected person. [.97]
2. Having an infected HIV person bite and break the skin. [.85]
3. Sharing of cigarettes, cigars, or pipes with an HIV infected person. [.87]
4. Uninfected person donating blood. [.87]
5. Receiving blood from an HIV infected person. [.98]
6. HIV infected mother to fetus.[.98]
7. HIV infected father to fetus. [.83]
8. Mosquitoes to person. [.86]
9. Lip kissing with an HIV infected person. [.88]
10. Tongue or "wet" kissing with an HIV infected person.[.85]
11. Sharing of eating utensils with an HIV infected person. [.81]
12. Sharing of toilet facilities with an HIV infected person. [.84]
13. Sharing of razors with an HIV infected person.[.90]
14. Sharing of toothbrushes with an HIV infected person. [.89]
15. Sharing of beds, linen, pillows with an HIV infected person. [.99]
16. HIV infected mother's breast milk to infant.[.87]
17. Having tears of a person with HIV touch you.[.89]
18. Being sneezed upon by an HIV infected person. [.84]
19. Being coughed upon by an HIV infected person. [.99]
20. Being breathed upon by an HIV infected person. [.99]
21. Mouth of uninfected person to penis contact with an HIV infected person. [.92]
22. Mouth of uninfected person to vulva/vagina contact with an HIV infected person. [.90]
23. Mouth of uninfected person to anus contact with an HIV infected person. [.85]
24. Anal intercourse with an HIV infected person. [.84]
25. HIV infected male to male intercourse. [.99]
26. HIV infected male to female intercourse. [.98]
27. HIV infected female to male intercourse. [.99]
28. HIV infected female to female sexual intimacies. [.82]
29. Male to animal intercourse. [.80]
30. Animal to male intercourse. [.81]
31. Female to animal intercourse. [.83]
32. Animal to female intercourse. [.85]
33. CPR instruction on manikins infected with HIV. [.80]

34. CPR on actual humans infected with HIV. [.86]
35. Being "spitted" upon by an HIV infected person. **
36. HIV infected patient to medical worker from a needlestick. [.84]
37. Patient receiving injections from medical workers. [.80]
38. Swimming in a pool with a person infected with HIV. [.98]

The following statements are either true or false. Mark A if true, mark B if false.

39. A good significant way to reduce your chances of "catching" the AIDS virus is for both partners to remain faithful to each other and not use I.V. drugs. [.99]
40. The more sexual partners a person has, the greater the risk of "catching" the AIDS virus. [.87]
41. A positive HIV antibody test means you have AIDS. [.87]
42. A positive HIV antibody test means you have been exposed to the virus. [.96]
43. HIV can be transmitted even if the person lacks symptoms. [.91]
44. Most babies born with the AIDS virus develop natural immunities, thus they can live a normal life. [.89]
45. Less than 1% of pregnant women with HIV transmit the disease to the fetus.[.82]
46. Many HIV transmissions have occurred among children in the school setting. [.95]
47. The contraction of the AIDS virus can be prevented or reduced significantly if a person abstains from sexual intercourse. [.82]
48. Most HIV infected individuals have become infected by using I.V. drugs. [.87]
49. Vaginal sex is more likely to spread the AIDS virus than anal sex. [.83]
50. The contraction of the AIDS virus can be prevented or reduced significantly by using a condom. [.98]
51. There have been a few reported cases of blood donors becoming infected with HIV while donating their blood. **
52. The contraction of the AIDS virus can be prevented or reduced significantly by having the male withdraw his penis just before ejaculation. [.80]
53. AIDS can be cured by large doses of antibiotics. [.96]
54. If one does not engage in certain "high risk" behaviors, there is almost no chance of contracting the AIDS virus. [.96]
55. The AIDS virus can remain infective in dried blood for several hours out of the body. [.82]
56. Nobody under 18 years of age has died of AIDS. [.88]

** Correlations below .80; statement has been rephrased; data on 60 subjects show reliability on revised statements to be .88 and .90 respectively.

4

THE ROLE OF SEXUAL ACTIVITY ON ADOLESCENT ATTITUDES: IMPLICATIONS FOR SEX EDUCATION PROGRAMS

Vivien C. Carver
Mark J. Kittleson
Ella P. Lacey

The purpose of this study was to determine the role of sexual activity in sexual knowledge, and attitudes. The subjects were 312 black high school students from a rural public school district in a Southern state. Subjects were administered Kirby's Sex Knowledge, Attitudes and Behaviors Scale. Overall, 70% of the subjects reported being non-virgin, while 87% of the males reported being non-virgin compared to 56% of the females. Tests of significance determined that statistically significant differences existed between virgins and non-virgins on numerous sexual attitudes. Discussion focused on identifying appropriate educational strategies related to these differences in attitudes.

It is estimated in the United States that 1.2 million females between the age of 15 and 19 become pregnant each year (Gilgun & Gordon, 1983; Rivara, Sweeney, & Henderson, 1985; Ventura, Taffel & Mosher, 1988). The results of these pregnancies produce various social and health concerns that affect all society. Ladner cites research that shows over 50% of teen mothers drop out of school directly because of pregnancy (Ladner, 1987). This problem is magnified in minority racial and ethnic populations that constitute 27% of all teens, yet account for 40% of teens who give birth annually (DiClemente, Boyer & Morales, 1988). In addition to concerns about pregnancy and its effects, there is concern about the growing risks associated with Human Immunodeficiency Virus (HIV) infection (Hardy & Duggan, 1988).

One of the major social concerns resulting from adolescent pregnancy is the loss of educational attainment opportunities which in turn often leads to economic deprivation (Moore, 1978). Society pays for this loss of work productivity in many ways, including lowered earning potential and lowered sense of self-esteem on the part of the female teen parent and her child/children (Card & Wise, 1978). However, social concerns are not limited to the pregnant teens (female) and their children, but also affect the adolescent fathers (males) who are 40% less likely to graduate from high school (Ladner, 1987; Moore, 1978), and are likely to suffer financial deprivation as well (Card & Wise, 1978; Hardy & Duggan, 1988).

In addition to the various social problems associated with adolescent pregnancies, there are cases where the health of both the mother and the child are at high risk. The health concerns with adolescent pregnancies for very young mothers have been well documented in low-birth weight of the fetus and its complications (Vanlandingham et al., 1988), as well as serious consequences to both the child and the mother from poor pre-natal and post neo-natal care (Black & DeBlassie, 1985).

Because of both health and social concerns, numerous sex education programs have been initiated. Questions arise over the goal of many of these programs - is it merely to inform about the "basic plumbing," or to elicit behavior change (i.e., to reduce adolescent pregnancies)? The ramifications of adolescent pregnancies overwhelmingly justify the need for encouraging behavior change. Trussell (1988) claims that reducing adolescent pregnancies should take priority over reducing adolescent sexual involvement. Regardless of the goal, it is apparent that merely teaching anatomy and physiology is ineffective in reducing adolescent pregnancies, sexual involvement, or the spread of sexually transmitted diseases. Unfortunately, many programs still teach only anatomy and physiology of the reproductive system, a reflection of the universally accepted belief that knowledge will directly affect attitude, which in turn will change behavior (Iverson & Portnoy, 1977). In general, this theory assumes that a person who knows which behaviors are inappropriate or risky will avoid such practice (Fischhoff, 1988; Swanson, 1972). The causal relationship between knowledge, attitudes/beliefs, and behaviors is weak (Kiesler & Kiesler, 1969). Bartlett's (1981) research supports the concept that health information programs tend to promote only knowledge change, with minimum behavior change.

When one reviews what is currently being taught in sex education, it is not unusual to see the emphasis on the teaching of "facts." In addition, most sexuality programs tend to focus on national norms and may not be appropriate for various sub-cultures and/or high-risk groups (Melchert & Burnett, 1989). It also appears that the neglect in current sex education programs does not take into account specific areas of differences between the virgins and non-virgins, especially in minority populations or high-risk groups (Melchert & Burnett, 1990).

Since it appears that sex education programs emphasizing the cognitive domain have failed in changing behavior, it may be time to emphasize other strategies. Some researchers endorse the concept of reversing the knowledge-attitude-behavior model (Parcel, 1985; Thompson, Daugherty, & Carver, 1984). One of those strategies would involve determining the role that current sexual behavior plays in sexual knowledge and attitudes. Therefore, the purpose of this study was to determine if the level of sexual activity plays a significant role in determining sexual attitudes. These findings could provide essential support for developing appropriate educational programs.

METHODOLOGY

The subjects were 312 black high school students from a predominately rural public school district in a southern state. The subjects who volunteered to participate in the study (181 females, 131 males) were selected from the two high schools in the school district. There were 121 tenth graders, 110 eleventh graders, and 81 twelfth graders (Table 1). Prior to the study, all subjects had completed a one-semester health education class in the tenth grade, which had included a unit on family life. Three homerooms from each grade level were randomly selected. The subjects who chose to participate were insured anonymity. The instrument was completed during a regular class period.

Permission was obtained from the superintendent and all participating principals in the school district to conduct the study. The instrument was administered by the researchers, who explained terminology and assisted with any problems.

Kirby's (1984) instrument on knowledge, attitudes, and behaviors was used. The test-retest reliability for this instrument was .89 for the knowledge test, and .51 to .88 for the attitude scale. The instrument consisted of: (1) a sex knowledge test of 30 multiple choice questions; (2) one behavioral question, which asked whether the subject had or had not ever engaged in sexual intercourse; and (3) an attitude scale with 47 items based on a 5-point Likert scale (strongly disagree to strongly agree). The attitudes were broken into the following sections:

A) Attitudes Toward Premarital Intercourse
B) Clarity of Personal Sexual Values
C) Attitudes Toward Sexuality in Life
D) Attitudes Toward the Use of Pressure and Force in Sexual Activity
E) Understanding Personal Sexual Response
F) Clarity of Long Term Goals
G) Satisfaction with Personal Sexuality
H) Importance of Birth Control

Frequencies and percentages were calculated for the subjects' response on the behavioral scale question. Analysis of variance was used in comparing the sexual behavior, grade level, and sex knowledge of the subjects. Chi-square was used to determine if significant differences existed in attitudes toward sex between the virgins and non-virgins. Significance levels were set at .05.

RESULTS

Sexual Behavior

The subjects were asked if they had ever engaged in sexual intercourse. This was the only behavioral question that was permitted by the superintendent and the school system. Those answering *yes* were considered to be non-virgins, whereas those answering *no* were classified as virgins. Seventy percent of the subjects were *non-virgins,* and 30% were *virgins.* Eighty-seven percent of the males and 56% of the females reported being non-virgin.

Sex Knowledge

A comparison between students classified as virgins and non-virgins was made on the knowledge test. An ANOVA revealed no significant difference between the two groups at the .05 level. The mean for all subjects on the knowledge test was 42.45%, indicating a general lack of sex knowledge (Table 1). This tends to contradict the Reichelt and Werley study that determined non-virgins were more knowledgeable than virgins (Reichelt & Werley, 1978).

A comparison between grade level and knowledge test scores was also made. The Davis and Harris study concluded that subjects who were older scored higher on sex knowledge (Davis & Harris, 1982). Table 2 indicates that a significant difference exists between the knowledge of 10th-, 11th-, and 12th-grade students. The Tukey's Post Hoc Analysis of multiple comparisons indicated that a significant difference (.05) in knowledge scores existed only between the 11th- and 12th-grade levels, somewhat contradicting Davis and Harris. Perhaps, as Bartlett indicated (1981), the recent completion of a one-semester health course (with a cognitive emphasis) could account for the fact that tenth graders outscored the 11th graders.

Attitudes Toward Sex

A second comparison was made between the virgins and non-virgins on the Kirby sex attitude scale. Kirby's sex attitude scale has 14 sections, with an underlying theme in each section. Because of the sensitivity of the questionnaire and the conservative nature of the administrators in this particular school system, only eight sections could be used for this study. One of the limitations of this study is that a factor analysis was not performed on the instrument. However, it is felt by the researchers that the results can still provide a valuable contribution to the field of health education. Chi-square was used to determine a statistically significant difference on 19 of the 47 attitudes. It is interesting to note that 15 of these attitudes were significant at the .01 level, and the remaining four were significant at the .05 level.

When analyzing these 19 significant attitudes, of special interest were the diametrically opposing viewpoints of the two groups. Virgins supported the following attitudes more strongly than the non-virgins:

Attitudes Toward Premarital Intercourse

1. Unmarried people should not have sex (29.6% virgins agreed compared to 18.9% non-virgins)
2. People should have sex before marriage (35.8% virgins agreed compared to 14.3% non-virgins)
3. People should have sex only if they are married (39.2% virgins agreed compared to 16.6% non-virgins)

Clarity of Personal Sexual Values

1. I'm confused about my sexual values and beliefs (22.9% virgins agreed compared to 17.9% non-virgins)
2. I'm confused about what I should/should not do sexually (40.2% virgins agreed compared to 24.4% non-virgins)

Attitudes Toward Sexuality in Life

1. Sexual relationships create more problems than they're worth (50% virgins agreed compared to 42.4% non-virgins)
2. Sexual relationships make life too difficult (23.9% virgins agree compared to 17.5% non-virgins)

Attitudes Toward the Use of Pressure and Force in Sexual Activity

1. A person should not pressure someone into sexual activity (79.3% virgins agreed compared to 77.4% non-virgins)
2. People should not pressure others to have sex with them (74% virgins agreed compared to 61.7% non-virgins)

Understanding Personal Sexual Response

1. When I'm in a sexual situation, I get confused about my feelings (30.5% virgins agreed compared to 28.6% non-virgins)

The non-virgins supported the following attitudes more strongly than virgins:

Attitudes Toward the Use of Pressure and Force in Sexual Activity

1. People should never take no for an answer when they want sex (37.3% non-virgins agreed compared to 20.7% virgins)
2. It is all right to pressure someone into sexual activity (22.3% non-virgins agreed compared to 6.5% virgins)
3. It is all right to demand sex from a boy/girlfriend (30.4% non-virgins agree compared to 14.1% virgins)

Understanding of Personal Sexual Response

1. I have a good understanding of my own sexual feelings and reactions (79.8% non-virgins agreed compared to 54.3% virgins)
2. I know how I react in different sexual situations (71.4% non-virgins agreed compared to 45.6% virgins)

Attitude Toward Sexuality in Life

1. A sexual relationship is one of the best things a person can have (54.9% non-virgins agreed compared to 18.5% virgins)
2. Sexual relationships provide an important and fulfilling part of life (65.3% non-virgins agreed compared to 41.3% virgins)

Attitude Toward Premarital Intercourse

1. It is all right for two people to have sex before marriage (70.1% non-virgins agreed compared to 56.5% virgins)

Clarity of Long Term Goals

1. I have a good idea of where I'm headed in the future (76% non-virgins agreed compared to 72.8% virgins)

DISCUSSION AND IMPLICATIONS
FOR SEX EDUCATORS

For a number of reasons, sex education programs tend to focus primarily on the cognitive aspects of sexuality. The premise seems to be to increase knowledge, so that attitudes and behaviors can be modified. If the rate of teenage pregnancy is any indication of the success of this program, it becomes clear that different approaches need to be considered. So pervasive is the belief that increased knowledge will have an impact on attitudes and behaviors that there has not been a great deal of research in examining the impact that sexual behavior has on sexual attitudes. This research made the explicit examination of the effect of sexual practice on sexual knowledge and attitudes, specifically in a black population. Obviously, this study needs to be replicated in order to confirm that these results are applicable to a broader population.

It is important to note that the sexual knowledge level of this population was low. Students correctly answered between 39 to 46% of the knowledge questions. This indicates that a one-semester course in health cannot provide adequate cognitive information on sexuality, let alone provide time necessary to focus on attitudes and decision-making. However, it is important to note that norms were established that can be of importance for those individuals involved in rural educational settings.

A second area of interest is the fact that 70% of the subjects were non-virgins. Again, this reiterates what we already know regarding adolescent sexual behavior. Obviously, this behavior lends itself to a number of social and health problems, including pregnancy and the acquisition of various sexually transmitted diseases.

The major focus of this study was to examine the differences in attitudes between those individuals who are classified as virgins and non-virgins. Such differences included the sub-category of: attitudes toward premarital intercourse, use of force to have sexual intercourse, clarity of personal sexual values, understanding personal sexual response, clarity of long term goals, and sexuality in life. Each issue has societal implications. The attitudes in the section on the use of force have significant impact on certain topics such as rape (including date rape), responsibility for adolescent pregnancies, transmission of HIV and other sexually transmitted diseases, as well as a host of other social problems. The fact that non-virgins have major differences in their attitudes on the use of force indicates to the health educator that such an issue needs to be discussed. Therefore, these attitudes have implications for the affective domain of sex education programs.

For example, regarding use of force, the non-virgins more strongly supported the attitude that one "...should never take no for an answer when they want sex," while the virgins were significantly less likely to agree. In addition to providing cognitive information, it may be appropriate for the classroom instructor or facilitator to include discussion of these statements and have the students analyze personal and societal consequences of such behavior, as well as the negating rationale. Such an approach has often been omitted or has been subject to varying interpretations.

The results also show that virgins tend to be more "confused" about personal sexual values than non-virgins. Discussing the importance and impact of being a sexual being should have an "affective" component. This study reveals those who are sexually active feel more confident about themselves.

Finally, it appears that those who are not sexually active have very different opinions about the role of premarital intercourse. Such information can be of value when discussing whether adolescents should become sexually involved.

CONCLUSION

With current concern regarding adolescent pregnancies and their many ramifications, especially among the black population, it is imperative for health educators to assist in developing culturally sensitive and appropriate educational programs. To attempt to reach a goal of reducing adolescent pregnancies by affecting adolescent sexual behavior, further study is needed to clarify differences in attitudes between the sexually active and the sexually non-active. Our study provides support for the idea that there may be differences in sexual knowledge and attitudes that should be incorporated into sex education programs. If sex education is expected to affect adolescent behaviors, then new approaches must be developed, implemented, and evaluated. It is hoped that this study will provide some impetus for health educators to initiate more research that attempts to understand adolescents and their inter-relationships as they affect sexual behaviors.

REFERENCES

Bartlett, E.E. (1981). The contribution of school health education to community health promotion: What can we realistically expect? *American Journal of Public Health, 71,* 1384-1391.

Black, C., & DeBlassie, R. (1985). Adolescent pregnancy: Contributing factors, consequences, treatment and plausible solutions. *Adolescence, 20,* 281-290.

Card, J., & Wise, L. (1978). Teenage mothers and teenage fathers: The impact of early childbearing on the parents' personal and professional lives. *Family Planning Perspectives, 10,* 199-205.

Davis, S.M., & Harris, M.B. (1982). Sexual knowledge, sexual interests and sources of sexual information of rural and urban adolescents from three cultures. *Adolescence, 17,* 471-491.

DiClemente, R.J., Boyer, C.B., & Morales, E.S. (1988). Minorities and AIDS: Knowledge, attitudes, and misconceptions among Black and Latino adolescents. *American Journal of Public Health, 78,* 55-57.

Fischhoff, B. (1988). Decision making on AIDS. Invited paper presented at the Vermont Conference on Primary Prevention, Burlington, VT. Sept.

Gilgun, J., & Gordon, S. (1983). The role of values in sex education programs. *Journal of Research and Development in Education, 16,* 27-33.

Hardy, J., & Duggan, A. (1988). Teenage fathers and the fathers of infants of urban, teenage mothers. *American Journal of Public Health, 78,* 919-922.

Iverson, D., & Portnoy, B. (1977). Reassessment of the knowledge/attitude/behavior triad. *Health Education, 8,* 31-34.

Kiesler, C.A., & Kiesler, S.B. (1969). *Conformity.* Reading, MA: Addison Wesley.

Kirby, D. (1984). *Sexuality education: A handbook for the evaluation of programs.* Santa Cruz, CA: Network Publications.

Ladner, J. (1987). Black teenage pregnancy: A challenge for educators. *Journal of Negro Education, 56,* 53-63.

Melchert, T., & Burnett, K.F. (1990). Attitudes, knowledge, and sexual behavior of high risk adolescents: Implications for counseling and sexuality education. *Journal of Counseling and Development, 68,* 293-298.

Moore, K. (1978). Teenage childbirth and welfare dependency. *Family Planning Perspectives, 10,* 233-235.

Parcel, G. (1985). Comments from the field. *Journal of School Health, 55,* 345-346.

Reichelt, P.A., & Werley, H.H. (1978). Sex knowledge of teenagers and the effects of an educational rap session. *Journal of Research and Development in Education, 10,* 13-22.

Rivara, F.P., Sweeney, P.J., & Henderson, B.F. (1985). A study of low socioeconomic status, black teenage fathers and their nonfather peers. *Pediatrics, 75,* 648-656.

Swanson, J.C. (1972). Second thoughts on knowledge and attitude effects upon behavior. *Journal of School Health, 42,* 363-365.

Thompson, M.L., Daugherty, R., & Carver, V.C. (1984). Alcohol education in schools: Toward a lifestyle risk-reduction approach. *Journal of School Health, 54,* 79-83.

Trussell, J. (1988). Teenage pregnancy in the United States. *Family Planning Perspectives, 20,* 262-272.

Vanlandingham, M.J., Buehler, J.W., Hogue, C.J.R., & Strauss, L.T. (1988). Birthweight-specific infant mortality for native Americans compared with whites, six states, 1980. *American Journal of Public Health, 78,* 499-505.

Ventura, S.J., Taffel, S.M., & Mosher, W.D. (1988). Estimates of pregnancies and pregnancy rates for the United States 1976-1985. *American Journal of Public Health, 78,* 506-511.

Table 1: Student Sexual Knowledge by Behavior

Group	n	Mean	SD	F	Sign
Virgin	92	44.18	18.59	1.23	NS
Non-Virgin	219	41.72	17.53		

* 3 subjects did not complete the sexual activity question

Table 2: Student Knowledge by Grade Level

Group	n	Mean	SD	F	Sign
Tenth Grade	121	43.00	16.46	3.76	Sign.
Eleventh Grade	110	39.00	17.95		
Twelfth Grade	81	46.00	19.01		

* Significant p < .05 between 11th Graders and 12th Graders

5

SPECIFIC SEX EDUCATION TOPIC INSTRUCTION TIME

Michael R. Davey

The purpose of this study was to investigate the amount of time spent teaching selected sex education topics in Illinois public schools. The topics investigated were anatomy and physiology, pregnancy, contraception, sexually transmitted disease, decision-making, and relationships. A ten percent proportionate stratified random sample technique was utilized to choose subjects. The existing Illinois State High School football classification system served as the stratification vehicle. The appropriate number of high schools was randomly selected from each class. After selection, schools that fed students (elementary, middle school, junior high) into each high school were included in the sample. The total number of schools was equal to 342. Of this total figure, 267 or 78% returned questionnaires. Responding school principals were instructed to indicate the amount of instruction time for each selected topic per grade level (K-3, 4-6, 7-8, 9-12, SPED). Further categorization by grade level yielded 525 cases. It was found that total mean hours of instruction per topic was minimal throughout both school size and grade level (total X = 4.90 hours). This investigation suggested that very little instruction time was devoted to formal sex education in Illinois public schools.

American children have inherited the worst of all possible worlds regarding their exposure to messages about sex. The media tells them that sex is romantic, exciting, and titillating, yet parents and church tell them to say no (Scales, 1987). And almost nothing that young people see or hear about sex informs them about contraception or the importance of avoiding pregnancy. Prime time television, regarded as at least second in importance to parents as a source of sexual influence, portrays sex mainly through innuendos and contextual references to intercourse (Gordon, 1986). For example, 89% of TV sex occurs outside of marriage and frequently is not presented as caring, loving, or considerate (Strouse & Fobes, 1985). This creates a mind set that sex is unidimensional or an overwhelming and uncontrollable physical attraction and desire devoid of responsibility.

American teenagers are becoming sexually active at younger ages (Hayes, 1988; Stark, 1986; Stout & Rivara, 1989). Surveys have shown that during the 1970s, the number of sexually active teens increased by approximately 66% over previous decades (Hayes, 1988; Hofferth et al., 1987; Sawyer & Beck, 1988; Stark, 1986). Among the 15 to 17 year olds in this country, 50% of the boys and 33% of the girls have experienced sexual intercourse (Hayes, 1988; Starke, 1986). One poll (Wattleton, 1987) reported that 57% of teenagers were sexually active by age 17. In addition, 66% of teens never use contraception or use it poorly, a pattern that continues into the 20s (Scales, 1987).

Depending on the study, 80% to 90% of Americans favor sex education in the public schools (Guttmacher, 1989; Hayes, 1988; Time, 1986; Stark, 1986). However, although most school systems throughout the United States report offering sex education as a part of the curriculum (Guttmacher, 1989; Stout & Rivara, 1989; Time, 1986) and 60% to 75% of American students receive some type of sex education instruction before they graduate from high school (Guttmacher, 1989; Stark, 1986; Stout & Rivara, 1989), it is estimated that less than 10% of America's school children are exposed to a meaningful and comprehensive sex education program (Gordon, 1986; Guttmacher, 1989; Scales, 1987; Stout & Rivara, 1989; Strouse & Fobes, 1985).

METHODOLOGY

The *Survey of Sex Education Instruction*, sponsored by the Sex Education Task Force of the Illinois Chapter of the American Academy of Pediatrics, was developed, in part, to determine the amount of time spent in formal sex education instruction in Illinois public schools. Due to the diverse nature of Illinois (rural vs. urban) and to insure an adequate representation of all public schools, a 10% proportionate stratified random sample technique was utilized to choose subjects. The existing Illinois State High School Athletic Association (ISHSAA) football classification system served as the stratification vehicle (1A, 2A, 3A, 4A, 5A, 6A). This system was used because schools were already classified according to student population and the investigator felt that Illinois' diversity would be adequately represented. The appropriate number of high schools were randomly selected from each class (1A-21, 2A-8, 3A-8, 4A-8, 5A-10, 6A-9). After selection, schools that fed students (elementary, middle school, junior high) into each high school were included into the sample. Schools selected, per class, were: 1A-21, 2A-32, 3A-35, 4A-50, 5A-85, and 6A-119. The total number was 342. Out of this total figure, 267 or 78% returned questionnaires (1A-16, 2A-25, 3A-18, 4A-34, 5A-65, 6A-109). Further categorization by specific grade level produced 525 cases (K-3=197, 4-6=207, 7-8=78, 9-12=32, and SPED=11). The number of cases per grade per class are reported in Table 1.

Questionnaires were mailed to building principals who were instructed to indicate the amount of time allotted for teaching specific sex education topics per grade level. The specific sex education topics chosen were anatomy and physiology, pregnancy, contraception, sexually transmitted disease, decision making and relationships. These specific topics were selected because the sex education task force felt they represented the core components of a sex education curriculum.

RESULTS

Total hours per topic and total mean hours per topic are reported in Table 2. Although 71.4% of the schools surveyed indicated teaching sex education, it was evident from examination of individual questionnaires that a minimal amount of time was devoted to formal sex education instruction. This was particularly true for grades K-3 and 4-6. As is illustrated, total mean hours equaled 15.85. A 1982 national survey found that 75% of urban school districts reported offering sex education. However, most programs were short, with 75% lasting for less than 20 hours (Stout & Rivara, 1989). The author felt that the total mean hours (15.85) computed in the present study were deceptive because Decision Making (X=6.18) and Relationships (X=4.76) are integrated into other health related topics such as substance abuse. In other words, were these specific topics taught exclusively as part of a sex education unit or were they taught in conjunction with units throughout the school year? When Decision Making and Relationships were not included, total mean hours of instruction equaled 4.90 for the remaining topics. In addition, the instruction time devoted to specific topics was not consistent between school classification. This is illustrated in Tables 1 through 6.

Grades K-3

Mean instruction times per topic per class for grades K-3 are reported in Table 3. As is illustrated, except for Decision Making (X=7.15) and Relationships (X=3.83), grades K-3 did not devote much time to the remaining sex education topics (Pregnancy=.00028 hours).

Grades 4-6

Mean instruction times per topic per class are reported in Table 4. Total mean hours equaled 14.92. When Decision Making and Relationships were not included, total mean hours of instruction equaled 4.61 for the remaining topics. When individual topics were examined, the most mean hours were devoted to Decision Making (5.68). Class 5A schools taught the most mean hours of Decision Making (15.91) while class 2A schools taught the least (.66). The mean instruction time for Relationships was 4.62 hours. Class 5A schools taught the most mean hours of Relationships (13.70) while class 2A schools taught the least (.41). The mean instruction time for Anatomy and Physiology was 2.91 hours. Class 1A schools taught the most mean hours of Anatomy and Physiology (5.0) while class 4A schools taught the least (.33).

The mean instruction time for STD was 1.06 hours. Class 6A schools taught the most mean hours of STD (1.63) while class 4A schools taught the least (0). The mean instruction time for Contraception was .33 hours. Class 5A schools taught the most mean hours of Contraception (1.07) while class 2A and 4A schools taught the least (0). The mean instruction time for Pregnancy was .30 hours. Class 3A schools taught the most mean hours of Pregnancy (.65) while class 4A schools taught the least (0).

Grades 7-8

Mean instruction times per topic per class are reported in Table 5. Total mean hours equaled 16.47. Total mean hours computed without Decision Making and Relationships equaled 9.03. A national survey conducted by the Guttmacher Institute (1989) revealed that schools were teaching less than 12 hours of sex education in the seventh grade. Grade 7-8 Illinois public schools exceeded these findings when Decision Making and Relationships were included in the mean instruction hours. However, when the mean instruction time was computed for the remaining topics minus Decision Making and Relationships, grade 7-8 Illinois public schools fit into the less than 12 hour group. When individual topics were examined, the most mean hours were devoted to Relationships (3.80). Class 5A schools taught the most mean hours of Relationships (5.04) while class 4A schools taught the least (.66). The mean instruction time for Decision Making was 3.63 hours. Class 5A schools taught the most mean hours of Decision Making (5.41) while class 2A schools taught the least (.85). The mean instruction time for Anatomy and Physiology was 3.04 hours. Class 6A schools taught the most mean hours of Anatomy and Physiology (3.85) while class 2A schools taught the least (.50). The mean instruction time for STD was 2.09 hours. Class 5A schools taught the most mean hours of STD (3.04) while class 2A schools taught the least (.21). The mean instruction time for Contraception was 1.99 hours. Class 5A schools taught the most mean hours of Contraception (4.63) while class 2A schools taught the least (.07). The mean instruction for Pregnancy was 1.90

hours. Class 6A schools taught the most mean hours of Pregnancy (2.50) while class 2A schools taught the least (.14).

Grades 9-12

Mean instruction times per topic per class are reported in Table 6. Total mean hours equaled 38.71. Total mean hours when Decision Making and Relationships were not computed were 19.54. A national survey conducted by the Guttmacher Institute (1989) revealed that schools were teaching slightly more than 18 hours of sex education in the 12th grade. Grade 9-12 Illinois public schools exceeded these findings when Decision Making and Relationships were included in the mean instruction hours. However, when the mean instruction time was computed for the remaining topics minus Decision Making and Relationships, grade 9-12 Illinois public schools appeared to correlate with the national findings. It should be noted that the mean instruction times for the present study were calculated for grades 9 through 12. When individual topics were examined, the most mean hours were devoted to Relationships (11.04). Class 2A schools taught the most mean hours of Relationships (20.14) while class 3A schools taught the least (1.66). The mean instruction time for Decision Making was 8.12 hours. Class 4A schools taught the most mean hours of Decision Making (15.0) while class 1A taught the least (2.85). The mean instruction time for Anatomy and Physiology was 5.71 hours. Class 4A schools taught the most mean hours of Anatomy and Physiology (14.0) while class 3A schools taught the least (1.0). The mean instruction time for STD was 5.60 hours. Class 4A schools taught the most mean hours of STD (16.0) while class 3A schools taught the least (1.0). The mean instruction time for Contraception was 4.12 hours. Class 4A schools taught the most mean hours of Contraception (12.0) while class 3A schools taught the least (1.16). The mean instruction for Pregnancy was 4.09 hours. Class 4A schools taught the most mean hours of Pregnancy (10.0) while class 3A schools taught the least (1.0).

Special Education

Mean instruction times per topic per class are reported in Table 7. Total mean hours equaled 49.40. Total mean hours computed without Decision Making and Relationships equaled 25.81. SPED was difficult to interpret because (1) grade levels were often ambiguous, (2) only class 1A, 2A, 5A, and 6A schools reported teaching SPED sex education, and (3) there were only eleven cases that included SPED sex education out of a total of 525. As a result, the author felt that the findings were distorted. The mean instruction time for Relationships was 12.77 hours. Class 5A schools taught the most mean hours of Relationships (30.12) while class 2A schools taught the least (1.33). The mean instruction time for Decision Making was 10.81 hours. Class 5A schools taught the most mean hours of Decision Making (26.62) while class 2A schools taught the least (0). The mean instruction time for Contraception was 9.13 hours. Class 5A schools taught the most mean hours of Contraception (22.62) while class 2A schools taught the least (0). The mean instruction time for Anatomy and Physiology was 7.86 hours. Class 5A schools taught the most mean hours of Anatomy and Physiology (14.37) while class 2A schools taught the least (2). The mean instruction time for STD was 5.45 hours. Class 5A schools taught the most mean hours of STD (11.62) while class 2A schools taught the least (1.66). The mean instruction time for Pregnancy was 2.0 hours. Class 5A schools taught the most mean hours of Pregnancy (7.13) while class 2A schools taught the least (.50).

DISCUSSION

The results of this investigation tended to illustrate that the specific sex education topics of Anatomy and Physiology, Pregnancy, Contraception, and STDs receive minimal instruction time in Illinois public schools. The minimal instruction time is even more evident when topics are investigated by individual school size. The results also tended to illustrate that formal sex education instruction in Illinois public schools was comparable to the majority of programs throughout the United States (Gordon, 1986; Guttmacher, 1989; Scales, 1987; Stout & Rivara, 1989; Strouse & Fobes, 1985). When mean instruction time was computed per school size, class 5A schools tended to dominate grades 7-8 and SPED while class 4A schools tended to dominate grades 9-12. There are a number of possible explanations for the minimal amount of time devoted to formal sex education instruction in Illinois public schools. First, 59% of the schools surveyed reported teaching sex education as part of a health class or unit. This implies that sex education must compete with other health related topics for time. In addition, although comprehensive health education is mandated in Illinois, interpretation of the statues is left to local school district control resulting in a lack of consistency from one community to the next. In other words, "sex is something mentioned in a junior high or high school health class" (Hayes, 1988). Secondly, even though the majority of parents surveyed favors sex education in the public schools, sex education teachers report a lack of parental and community support (Guttmacher, 1989). In addition, school administrators often report feeling nervous about possible adverse community reaction to sex education (Guttmacher, 1989). Two other possibilities include difficulty in finding good, acceptable curriculums and debates on content and duration and perceived effectiveness in combating problems such as adolescent sexual activity and teen pregnancy.

In summary, the following patterns tended to emerge from this investigation:

1. A minimal amount of time was devoted to the specific sex education topics of Anatomy and Physiology, Pregnancy, Contraception and Sexually Transmitted Disease in Illinois public schools. The topics of Decision Making and Relationships appeared to receive adequate amounts of instruction time in Illinois public schools.

2. Formal sex education instruction appeared to be taught as part of a health education class or unit and was not comprehensive.

3. There was no consistent pattern of formal sex education instruction in Illinois public schools.

4. Classes 4A and 5A schools tended to devote the most amount of time to both specific sex education topics and formal sex education instruction.

REFERENCES

Gordon, S. (1986). What kids need to know. *Psychology Today,* October, 22-26.

Hayes, L. (1988). Critics agree sex education poor, clash over remedy. *Guidepost,* December 22, 3-5.

Hofferth, S., Kahn, J. & Baldwin, W. (1987). Premarital sexual activity among US teenage women over the past three decades. *Family Planning Perspectives, 19,* 46-50.

Sawyer, R. & Beck, K. (1988). Predicting pregnancy and contraceptive usage among college women. *Health Education, 19,* 42-47.

Scales, P. (1987). How we can prevent teen pregnancy and why it's not the real problem. *Journal of Sex Education Therapy, 13,* 12-15.

Sex and schools (1986). *Time,* November 24, 54-63.

Stark, E. (1986). Young, innocent, and pregnant. *Psychology Today,* October, 28-35.

Stout, J. & Rivara, R. (1989). Schools and sex education: Does it work? *Pediatrics, 83,* 375-379.

Strouse, J. & Fobes, R. (1985). Formal versus informal sources of sex education: Competing forces in the sexual socialization of adolescents. *Adolescence, 20,* 251-263.

The Alan Guttmacher Institute (1989). *Risk and responsibility: Teaching sex education in America's schools today.*

Wattleton, F. (1987). American teens: Sexually active, sexually illiterate. *Journal of School Health, 57,* 379-380.

Table 1

Number of Cases per Grade per Class

	K-3	4-6	7-8	9-12	SPED
1A	8	10	7	7	3
2A	16	18	7	7	3
3A	8	10	4	3	0
4A	25	21	6	2	0
5A	48	52	23	7	4
6A	92	95	31	6	1
Total	197	207	78	32	11

Table 2

Total Hours and Mean Hours per Topic

	Total Hours	Mean Hours
A&P	1104	2.11
Pregnancy	380	.72
Contraception	457	.83
STD	622	1.18
Decision Making	3235	6.18
Relationships	2494	4.76
Total	8292	15.85
*	2563	4.90

* = Total hours and total mean hours minus decision making and relationships.

Table 3

Grades K-3 Mean Instruction Time per Topic per Class

	1A	2A	3A	4A	5A	6A	Total
A&P	0	0	0	0	0	0	0
Preg.	0	0	0	0	.03	0	0
Contra.	0	0	0	0	0	0	0
STD	0	0	0	0	0	0	0
DM	.43	.75	37.50	.12	22.27	.22	7.15
REL	.87	.46	0	.04	14.89	.26	3.83
Total							10.98

Table 4

Grades 4-6 Mean Instruction Time per Topic per Class

	1A	2A	3A	4A	5A	6A	Total
A&P	5.0	.58	.95	.33	2.74	4.02	2.91
Preg.	.55	.05	.65	0	.31	.34	.30
Contra.	.44	0	.40	0	1.07	.05	.33
STD	.33	.77	.45	0	.95	1.63	1.06
DM	1.72	.66	15.65	1.33	15.91	1.31	5.68
REL	2.66	.41	.75	0	13.70	2.07	4.62
Total							14.92
*							4.61

* = Mean hours minus Decision Making and Relationships.

Table 5

Grades 7-8 Mean Instruction Time per Topic per Class

	1A	2A	3A	4A	5A	6A	Total
A&P	1.64	.50	1.06	2.83	3.36	3.85	3.04
Preg.	.42	.14	.87	1.66	2.32	2.50	1.90
Contra.	1.28	.07	1.50	1.00	4.63	.88	1.99
STD	1.50	.21	2.37	1.41	3.04	2.04	2.09
DM	2.57	.85	3.12	1.00	5.41	3.75	3.63
REL	1.71	.85	4.12	.66	5.84	3.98	3.80
Total							16.47
*							9.03

* = Total mean hours minus decision making and relationships.

Table 6

Grades 9-12 Mean Instruction Time per Topic per Class

	1A	2A	3A	4A	5A	6A	Total
A&P	2.00	6.50	1.00	14.00	7.07	7.16	5.71
Preg.	1.14	6.28	1.00	10.00	5.21	3.25	4.09
Contra.	2.85	4.14	1.16	12.00	4.92	3.50	4.12
STD	2.21	6.07	1.00	16.00	6.78	6.50	5.60
DM	2.85	10.28	3.50	15.00	9.57	10.08	8.12
REL	8.42	20.14	1.66	18.00	10.35	6.66	11.04
Total							38.71
*							19.54

* = Total mean hours minus decision making and relationships.

Table 7

SPED Mean Instruction Time per Topic per Class

	1A	2A	5A	6A	Total
A&P	6.66	2.00	14.37	3.00	7.86
Preg.	2.00	.50	7.12	1.00	3.36
Contra.	2.66	0	22.62	2.00	9.13
STD	2.00	1.66	11.62	2.50	5.45
DM	3.66	0	26.62	1.50	10.81
REL	4.66	1.33	30.12	2.00	12.77
Total					49.40
*					25.81

* = Total mean hours minus decision making and relationships.

6

ASSESSMENT OF COGNITIVE LEVEL TASK DEMANDS IN HIGH SCHOOL HEALTH EDUCATION CLASSES

David C. Wiley

The purpose of this study was to use quantitative methodology to describe the types of cognitive task demands placed upon students in high school health education classes. The importance of this pedagogical study was that the classroom processes were measured, as opposed to the more commonly observed "product" measures of student outcomes. Twenty high school health education teachers were observed on four occasions to assess their respective classroom activities. Prior to each observation, each teacher was interviewed as to his/her specific task demands on students for that lesson. The levels of Bloom's Taxonomy of Educational Objectives were used as the scale for interviewers to identify the cognitive task demands. The results were compiled across categories of task demands, as well as across each teacher by observation period. It was found that the knowledge level of task demand was reported on 33% of the observations. The next most commonly observed was a combination of task demands (i.e., knowledge with synthesis) 27% of the time. Synthesis was observed 15% of the time, while application was reported in 14% of the observations. Although knowledge was the most commonly observed task demand, teachers were found to use a variety of cognitive tasks across each of the four observations. By first employing descriptive studies, such as this study, the "process-product" model can be developed to provide important information as to the appropriate cognitive task demands needed for students in health education.

141

Research has indicated that comprehensive school health education does make a difference in promoting healthy lifestyles among adolescents. The School Health Program Evaluation study confirmed that optimally 50 hours of health instruction was required annually to maximally influence student knowledge, attitude, and behavior (Connell, Turner, & Mason, 1985).

However, the issue of quality health instruction remains a topic to be discussed. Merely conducting health education classes, without regard to the quality of instruction, could have a significant impact on the effectiveness of the school health education experience. Not only should research efforts target the "product" of student achievement, but the "process" of teaching should also be investigated. The "Process-Product" model is a valid tool which has been used in research on teaching in other content areas (Brophy & Good, 1986).

Gage (1985) has identified a process variable as anything that goes on in the classroom. This broad definition includes, but is not limited to, teacher behaviors, teaching styles, teaching methods, student behaviors, and teacher-student interaction. Fundamentally, the value in studying process variables is that they can be linked to product variables, such as test scores or student attitude scales.

Two health education classroom process studies have been reported. Hammonds and Schultz (1984) discovered that large group discussion was most often employed by teachers and preferred by students when teaching social and emotional aspects of sexuality. Educational media and guest speakers were the instructional techniques used and preferred to address physiological aspects of sexuality. Wiley, Peterson, and Silverman (1989) reported that high school education teachers used Teacher Presentation of Content (i.e., lecture) 23.4% of classroom time and Seatwork 23.1% of the time. Little classroom time was spent in Student Presentations (.3%).

One process variable which has yet to be investigated in health education settings is that of academic work. Academic work refers to the various task demands placed on students through the curriculum. To understand classroom processes, one must first understand the context in which the classroom functions. This contextual framework includes teacher and student perceptions of the task at hand (Berliner, 1983).

It has been observed that tasks link behavior with intention of purpose. Therefore, tasks provide a framework for interpreting what is said or done by the teacher in the classroom. Also, recurring activities in the classroom are shaped by task demands. Within this conceptualization, an interpretation of what is observed must be made within the context of the students' task demand. To merely know that the teacher asked a question does little to clarify the meaning of the question. The teacher's intent may be to have a student recall knowledge, jar that student from daydreaming, provide a opportunity for abstract thought, or begin a classroom discussion (Anderson, 1984).

Academic tasks are characterized by three aspects of students' work: (a) the products students are to formulate; (b) the operations used to generate the product; and (c) the resources available to students while they are generating a product (Doyle, 1983).

Therefore, the purpose of this process study was to describe the cognitive task demands placed on students in high school health education classes. By describing the cognitive level task demands used in these health education settings, future research can then focus on links to student achievement.

METHOD

Participants

Twenty high school health education teachers in a large southwestern city volunteered to have their classes studied during the spring of 1988. Though participants were volunteers, all secondary school health teachers (n=24) in the city were invited to participate. All health educators in the study taught at high schools with enrollments of at least 1000 students, with ten high schools being represented. Teaching experience for participants ranged from three to 28 years, with the average being 13.7 years. With the exception of one teacher, all participants were certified in health education by the Texas Education Agency. The average years of health education teaching experience was 7.6 years, with a range of one to 17 years.

Instrumentation and Data Collection

Each teacher agreed to have their respective classes observed on four separate class periods, on four separate days, yielding a total of 80 observations. Prior to each class period, the teacher was interviewed using the standardized Teacher Interview Form (Figure 1). Basic information was collected regarding the unit being covered and the topic for the day. Each teacher was also asked about the task demand for that day's lesson, the expected student outcomes for the lesson, and the resources available to the students to generate the desired outcome. Teachers were asked to describe the task for the day based upon descriptors from Bloom's Taxonomy of Educational Objectives (1956) (Figure 2). If the observer was unsure as to the exact focus of the lesson or if the teacher was ambiguous, additional descriptors were provided to the teacher regarding the levels of the taxonomy. No attempt was made to interpret or evaluate the task demand for the students, since the objective of the project was to describe these task demands.

RESULTS

The types of task demands placed on health education students are displayed in Table 1. The most common task demands involved the lowest level of Bloom's Taxonomy, knowledge. The majority of these knowledge task demands involved memorization of content-related definitions or terms. The second most prevalent task demands involved a combination of cognitive levels. Such levels typically included combining knowledge and synthesis, knowledge and application, and/or knowledge and comprehension.

Table 2 examines task demands as stated by the teacher across each of the four classroom observations. Although the knowledge level was the most commonly stated task demand on students, it should be noted that every teacher used a variety of task demands across the four observations. This finding highlights the point that the observed health education instructors varied their academic demands on students.

Teachers also reported that the products students were to generate were typically based on recall of factual information. Very little use of abstract thought was reported. In addition, the textbook was the primary resource available to students to generate the product. Although teachers used handouts and overheads, etc. the assist the students, the vast majority of these handouts and overheads were from the textbook or teacher's guide to the textbook.

DISCUSSION

In this study, the most commonly observed cognitive level was knowledge, the lowest level of Bloom's Taxonomy. While it is certainly important that students have a solid knowledge base in health education, health decisions involve much more than pure knowledge. According to the National Adolescent Student Health Survey (NASHS):

> It is clear from the findings of the study that knowledge is not all that is necessary for adolescents to make healthy choices. Education programs and interventions need to go beyond knowledge in order to address decision making and behavior. There needs to be explicit focus on sharpening students abilities to make decisions as well as a focus on helping students develop the personal desire to be a healthy individual (Dalis, 1988, pp. 2-3).

This concern that adolescents learn and practice critical thinking skills is heightened by the fact that the school health education program will be the only health education instruction which many adolescents will receive. Therefore, it is crucial that school health educators not only provide students with a good knowledge base, but that students are also given the opportunity to analyze and synthesize information related to good health decisions. Clearly, reading the textbook and taking tests over the material is not quality, comprehensive health instruction.

The results of this study might also have implications for university teacher training programs. University teaching "methods" courses should provide training to encourage higher-level thinking in the health education class. Student teachers should be required to go beyond textbook rote memorization and encouraged to try innovative teaching strategies designed to place students in realistic health decision scenarios. Such techniques would include, but are not limited to, values clarification exercises, group discussions, and role playing.

Although the results of this study may not apply universally to school health instruction, this study has highlighted the need for additional process studies in health education settings. Process studies, such as the one reported here, should be conducted in locales across the country to see if common health education teaching practices exist. Such studies would provide important information for establishing a baseline of common school health education teaching practices. Once these common practices are identified, correlational and experimental treatments could provide definitive information as to "effective" teaching practices using the process-product model.

As evidenced by the dearth of health education classroom studies, the school health classroom is one area in need of sustained research efforts. The "effectiveness" of many health education efforts are usually based on some special intervention for the adolescent population. Special intervention such as substance abuse or teenage pregnancy prevention programs typically include an evaluation component to provide measures of effectiveness. However, it would seem that the daily workings of the health education classroom would be of great interest to those interested in the health of adolescents. Although these special interventions can prove to be valuable, the day-to-day interactions of the school health program could provide crucial information as to curriculum needs and those teaching strategies which have a positive effect on student knowledge, attitude, and behavior.

REFERENCES

Anderson, L.W. (1984). Concerns for appropriate instrumentation in research on classroom teaching (Special Issue). *Evaluation in Education, 8(2)*.

Berliner, D.C. (1983). Developing conceptions of classroom environments: Some light on the T in classroom studies of ATI. *Educational Psychologist, 18(1)*, 1-13.

Brophy, J.E. & Good, T.L. (1986). Teacher behavior and student achievement. In M.C. Wittrock (Ed.), *Handbook of Research on Teaching* (pp. 328-375), New York: Macmillan.

Connell, D.B., Turner, R.R., & Mason, E.F. (1985). *School health education evaluation final report* (Vol. 1-4). Washington, D.C.: U.S. Department of Health and Human Services.

Dalis, G.T. (1988). National adolescent student health survey (NASHS). *Alliance Update*, 2-3.

Doyle, W. (1983). Academic work. *Review of Educational Research, 53(2)*, 159-199.

Gage, N.L. (1985). *Hard gains in the soft sciences: The case of pedagogy* (Phi Delta Kappa Monograph). Bloomington, IN: Center on Evaluation, Development, and Research.

Hammonds, M.M. & Schultz, J.B. (1984). Sexuality education instructional techniques: Teacher usage and student preference. *Journal of School Health, 54*, 235-238.

Wiley, D.C., Peterson, F.L., & Silverman, S.J. (1989). A descriptive analysis of activity structures in high school health education classes. *Journal of School Health, 59,* 393-397.

Figure 1

Teacher Interview Form

This interview should be conducted prior to every observation.

Teacher ID# (61)
Observation # (3)
Observers Initials (DCW)

1.   What is the unit being covered at this time? (i.e., first aid)

Nutrition

2.   What is today's topic? (i.e., controlling bleeding)

consumerism & buying habits

3.   What are the student outcomes expected as a result of today's lesson? (i.e., identify 3 methods for controlling bleeding)

Ss will id 5 advertising methods

4.   How are the students to generate this outcome? (i.e., memorizing lists or classifying concepts, etc.)

memorize & synthesize from lecture

5.   What resource will be available to students while they are generating the desired outcome? (i.e., finished models or diagrams, etc.)

examples of advertising will be presented by T using op

6. Are there any unusual routines, procedures, or activities in today's lesson?

   No

7. How are the students to be assessed on today's lesson?

   Ss will present "commercials" (designed by Ss) on advertising concepts

Figure 2

BLOOM'S TAXONOMY OF EDUCATIONAL OBJECTIVES (1956)

DOMAIN	DESCRIPTORS
1. KNOWLEDGE (K)	DEFINES, DESCRIBES, MEMORIZES
2. COMPREHENSION (C)	CONVERTS, DEFENDS, EXPLAINS
3. APPLICATION (A)	CHANGES, COMPUTES, MODIFIES
4. ANALYSIS (AN)	DIAGRAMS, DISCRIMINATES, INFERS
5. SYNTHESIS (S)	SUMMARIZES, COMBINES, COMPILES
6. EVALUATION (E)	CONCLUDES, INTERPRETS, CRITICIZES

Table 1

Frequency of Cognitive Level Task Demands
(n=80 observations)

Cognitive Level	Frequency	Percentage
1. Knowledge	26	33
2. Comprehension	1	0
3. Application	11	14
4. Synthesis	12	15
5. Combination of Levels	21	27
6. Other	9	11

Note: "Other" consists of those lessons when tests were given and/or the teacher had no student task demands for the lesson.

Table 2

Cognitive Task Demands by Instructor Across Observations

Teacher #	Observation #			
	1	2	3	4
1	S	K	K	K, A
2	S	S	O	A
3	K	A	K,A,S	K,S
4	S	K	A	K,A
5	S	A,S	O	K,S
6	K,S	K	K	K
7	K	A	K	K,A
8	K	K,S	K,S	K
9	K	K,A	K,S	K
10	S	K	K	K
11	K,S	K,S	A	S
12	K	S	O	K
13	K	O	K	K
14	O	A	S	A
15	O	K,S	K	K,C
16	O	S	S,A	A
17	K	K	O	S
18	O	S,A	A	K,C
19	C,S	A	K	S
20	C	K,A	A	K

K = Knowledge   C = Comprehension   A = Application
S = Synthesis   O = Other

Note: "Other" consists of those lessons when tests were given and/or the teacher had no student task demands for the lesson.

7

HEALTH EDUCATION PRIORITIES FOR ADOLESCENTS BY PHYSICIANS AND EDUCATORS: A MULTIDIMENSIONAL ANALYSIS

Murray A. Preston
Richard I. Evans
Phyllis M. Levenson-Gingiss

Traditional approaches to survey research regarding the selection of content for health promotion programs tend to view selection as a linear process. Since perceptions are often multidimensional in nature, methods of analysis must allow evaluation of the dynamics underlying selection. Four hundred fifty-one members of the Society for Adolescent Medicine and 329 members of the American School Health Association participated in a mail survey designed to ascertain their perceptions of the importance of including nine issues in school-based health promotion programs for adolescents and the extent to which issues selected as very important were perceived as similar to each other. Multidimensional scaling (MDS) was used to assess and compare the dimensions of the selection process and to determine if selection responses varied by professional affiliation. MDS analyses indicated agreement on the groups' perceptions of the similarities among issues. Sexual intercourse and substance abuse issues were most frequently designated by both groups as "very important" for inclusion. School Health respondents were more likely than Adolescent Medicine respondents to perceive nutritional, sexual, and marijuana use issues as "very important" for inclusion. Results are presented in terms of the implications of this approach for analyzing priority estimates of health professionals.

The selection of health issues for inclusion in health promotion programs targeted at young adolescents is a critical issue given the limits of time and funding available to reach this group. What is defined as a potential health problem may depend on who is being asked. The problems addressed in health education programs developed for adolescents are usually the problems attributed to the adolescents by the adults who plan the programs (Parcel, Nader & Mayer, 1977). The adults may be parents, teachers, public health officials, physicians, or others in health related fields. The perspective of these groups of adults varies because each is likely to encounter teens under different health or illness related circumstances (Levenson, Morrow & Pfefferbaum, 1984) and to have had a specialized rather than multidisciplinary focus to their professional training (Blum & Smith, 1988). Levenson and her colleagues (1984) emphasize that each of these groups has a unique contribution to make toward improving the health status of adolescents, but that seldom do the groups share or compare their views of the health related needs of this age group. Since the perceptions of health care providers influences their approach to certain adolescent health issues (Fortenberry, Kaplan & Hill, 1988), the factors influencing those perceptions require further examination.

The role of cognitions in generating behavior is the subject of debate. Ajzen and Fishbein (1973) and others (e.g., Hochbaum, 1973; Rosenstock, 1974) have proposed that behavior is a result of reasoned processes - multiple regression models of cognitive assessment to explain intention to behave which, in turn, is said to predict behavior. Yet there has been considerable discussion on the topic of how reasoned actions are, on the orderliness of the thought processes that precede behavior, and even on the ability of the individual to accurately report processes of thought that precede behavior (Alba & Hasher, 1983; Nisbett & Wilson, 1977; Tversky & Kahneman, 1974). These latter perspectives view cognition as multidimensional and hierarchically arranged, while possibly connected with the linear networks implied by a multiple regression model. Though perception, as a component of cognitive processes, is not viewed as causing behavior, it is viewed as a mediator of behavior, and the study of perception allows evaluation of the bases of behavior. Thus one would expect to gather different, though complementary, information by exploring cognitive processes that underlie behavior from a multidimensional perspective than by exploring from a more linear perspective. Considering the present discussion, the multidimensional perspective would precede the more linear representation in the process of making judgements.

Surveys employing fixed alternative and/or open-ended items are a widely used methodology in the needs assessment phase of health promotion programs. Previously, the selection of health issues to be addressed in adolescent health promotion programs has been examined in terms of pre-intervention surveys to determine who has selected the health issues (e.g., Parcel et al., 1977), which issues should be considered the focus of the selection process (e.g., Iverson & Kolbe, 1983), and which issues have been selected (e.g., Dratt & Evans, 1985; Levenson, Morrow, Morgan & Pfefferbaum, 1986). Dratt (1985) examined the extent to which the selection process was influenced by question format. While he found that open-ended questions regarding the selection of health issues elicited different priorities for health education content than selection of health issues from lists provided to the respondent, the perceptual basis for these priorities was not explored. In general, these studies have approached decisions related to health behavior from a linear, reasoned process, perspective.

The present paper explores the application of Multidimensional Scaling (MDS) in a survey regarding the selection of health education priorities for adolescents. It extends the process of selecting health program content to allow for identification of the multidimensional nuances of cognition which underlie the selection of health issues. In the present paper the authors present one example of a means of identifying more subtle cognitive components than is possible through traditional survey research methodology.

The study compares responses from members of two professional organizations, the Society for Adolescent Medicine and the American School Health Association. The Society for Adolescent Medicine consists primarily of pediatricians whose practice emphasizes the promotion of adolescent health. Members of the American School Health Association are primarily nurses and health educators who have specialized in the promotion of health in school settings. Two aspects of respondents' views of nine health issues were examined: (1) which issues were selected as "very important" for inclusion in health promotion programs for adolescents, and (2) the extent to which issues selected as very important were perceived as similar to each other.

It was hypothesized that those in the two professional organizations would differ both in their assessment of the importance of health issues for inclusion in health promotion programs and in their perceptions of the health issues as similar to each other. The proposed bases for these differences were (1) the professional training of the two groups which may influence them to approach similar issues from different perspectives, and (2) the health or illness-related circumstances under which the two groups encounter teens (Levenson et al., 1984). The utility of using MDS techniques to examine these issues will be assessed.

METHODS

Subjects

The membership of the Society for Adolescent Medicine (SAM) and a stratified random sample of the American School Health Association (ASHA) received a survey instrument by mail. The total sample consisted of all members of SAM (880), and 986 members of ASHA. Response rates were 51% and 33%, respectively.

Questionnaire

A three part survey instrument was developed for use in the present study (available upon request). The first section contained nine items taken from a more comprehensive questionnaire of 30 items, originally used by Dratt (1985). Items in Dratt's questionnaire were rated by teachers and parents of adolescents in terms of their importance for inclusion in a health promotion program targeted at 7th to 9th graders. The rating categories were *Very Unimportant, Unimportant, Neither Important Nor Unimportant, Important,* and *Very Important.* Items were selected for the present study in a two stage process. First, the 30 health issues were ranked by mean importance rating. Then, three items each from the high, middle, and low range were selected for the present study. Selected items were as follows:

How important is it for 7th to 9th graders to learn to
-care for skin properly
-eat healthy food
-handle pressures to sniff paint, glue, or other substances
-handle pressures to use drugs such as amphetamines, barbiturates, hallucinogens
-report and get help for child abuse
-handle pressures to smoke cigarettes
-refuse to ride with drivers who are or have been drinking
-handle pressures to engage in sexual intercourse
-handle pressure to use the drug marijuana

Three of these items (drugs, marijuana, sex) were rated as very important for inclusion; three items (nutrition, drunk driving, cigarettes) were rated in the middle range; and three items (child abuse, inhalants, skin care) had the lowest importance ratings for inclusion in a health promotion program for adolescents. This hierarchy of ratings is an important part of the present study, since to use Multidimensional Scaling analysis, the stimuli must vary sufficiently on an associated attribute for dimensions to appear (Kruskal & Wish, 1978). These health issues were selected because of variations in their perceived importance and were not meant to be inclusive of all adolescent health concerns.

The second section of the survey consisted of 36 items. It was developed to allow for analysis of these data utilizing Multidimensional Scaling (MDS) with the INDSCAL option specified. An example from the second section of the questionnaire follows:

EXAMPLE:

Failing to care for   Having unhealthy
skin properly   eating habits
IDENTICAL   0   1   2   3   4   5   6   7   8   9   DIFFERENT

If you feel that these behaviors are similar to each other in terms of their long term effects on the health and safety of 7th to 9th grade teenagers in general, then you would circle a number closer to the word IDENTICAL to show how similar you consider them to be.

If you feel that these behaviors are different from each other in terms of their long term effects on the health and safety of 7th to 9th grade teenagers in general, then you would circle a number closer to the word DIFFERENT to show how different you consider them to be.

Respondents were asked to rate on the ten point interval scale, all possible nonduplicating pairs of the nine health issues, on the extent to which they are identical or different.

MDS is a class of statistical techniques which uses proximities of any kind of objects as input, and which provides as output, a spatial representation intended to reveal the underlying cognitive structure of the proximity ratings (Kruskal & Wish, 1978; Schiffman, Reynolds & Young, 1981; Subkoviak, 1975). Uses for MDS have included applications as varied as the measurement of cognitive mapping techniques regarding the physical location of stimuli such as cities in the United States, and of qualities of taste regarding consumer products prior to marketing efforts. In the present study, this utility was extended to the measurement of respondents' cognitive appraisal of the similarity of health behaviors in terms of their long term effects on the health and safety of 7th to 9th graders. INDSCAL allows individual proximity ratings to be used to generate a measure of how important the arrangement of objects in a configuration is to the perceptions of each subject (Schiffman et al., 1981); an average of these weights gives an indication of the overall importance of each dimension to the perceptions of the total sample of respondents. The use of identical and different rather than other attributes more directly related to health beliefs is an integral part of the MDS technique (Schiffman et al., 1981), which allows the researcher to discover rather than to impose the dimensions on which the perceptual spacing is based (Kruskal & Wish, 1978). The level of agreement of the original similarity ratings with the multidimensional configuration is evaluated by two indices of goodness of fit. One index is the value associated with stress in fitting the data to the configuration. This indicates the degree to which the data had to be forced or stressed in order to produce the configuration. A second index of goodness of fit is r^2, the proportion of variance accounted for by the solution (Schiffman et al., 1981).

Data from this section was analyzed, using ALSCAL-4, INDSCAL option (Young & Lewyckyj, 1981) a multidimensional scaling (MDS) package available through the Statistical Analysis System (SAS). The spatial display which results from the MDS analysis consisted of a geometric configuration of points, each of which corresponded to one of the nine health issues. Both the arrangement of health issues along two dimensions and the grouping of health issues within the configuration were analyzed in terms of their proximity to each other. As suggested by Kruskal and Wish (1978), the data for each professional organization was split into two groups and the groups were analyzed separately to assess the reliability of the geometric representations produced by the analyses. This was accomplished by analyzing the data from odd and then even-numbered subjects separately.

While some consider the number of dimensions to be only limited by stress value, r^2, and interpretability (Schiffman et al., 1981; Smith, Falvo, McKillip, & Pitz, 1984), Subkoviak (1975) cautions that the number of possible dimensions should be limited by the number of stimulus items. The present study used nine stimulus items in the form of health issues. Following Subkoviak, this limits interpretability to a two-dimensional solution, with goodness of fit indicated by stress values and r^2. This limitation on the maximum number of dimensions was stipulated in the format of the MDS program. Within this limitation MDS recovered the underlying structure among the health issue stimuli.

The second section of 36 items allowed examination of the underlying perceptual dimensions of the proximity ratings of the nine items from the first section of the survey instrument.

The third section gathered demographic information about the respondents. Where it was practical, this section used the same response categories as those used by SAM and ASHA in their membership information forms. Additionally, in the case of SAM, this section was designed to assist the society in gathering information about their membership.

The survey instrument was pretested by five pediatricians and twelve school health educators for clarity and readability. The investigators used feedback from the pretest to reformat the instrument. Each survey instrument was accompanied by a letter on the letterhead of the respective professional organization. The letter explained that the organization was sponsoring the survey of its members, emphasized that participation was voluntary, and asked each member to participate. The letter, survey, and a postage-paid return envelope were mailed in envelopes generally used by SAM and ASHA. Four weeks later, a second set of survey instruments was mailed. This mailing was identical to the first with two exceptions: The survey instrument had a later requested date of return, and the envelope included an additional letter asking members to respond if they had not already done so.

RESULTS

Description of Respondents

Society for Adolescent Medicine. The 470 respondents from SAM represented approximately 55% of the total membership. Of this total, 19 instruments could not be analyzed because of insufficient data. The remaining 451 survey instruments, representing 51% of the membership, were analyzed. Further description of the SAM subjects will refer to these 451 respondents.

Sixty-four percent of respondents were male, and 36% were female. Approximately 65% of the respondents were between the ages of 30 and 49. Congruent with the relative youth of this group, approximately 55% of the respondents had completed their formal training within the ten years immediately prior to their participation in the study. Physicians represented 89% of the respondents; 4% were nurses; 2% were psychologists; and 5% specified professions such as social work, health education, health administration, sociology and nutrition. Forty-eight percent of the physicians either had completed or were completing a formal fellowship in Adolescent Medicine.

Thirty-four percent of respondents worked in an academic setting, 29% had a private practice, 23% worked in a combination of academic and private practice, while 13% described their work settings as clinical/non-private practice. A remaining 2% did not specify their work setting. Eighty percent of respondents worked in urban areas. Rural and mixed (urban and rural) made up the location of 14% and 6% of respondents' work locations, respectively. The survey focused on health issues with respect to 7th to 9th graders. The practice of 42% of the respondents included less than 25% of this age group; for 43% of respondents, their practice included 26-50% 7th to 9th graders; an additional 11% estimated that 51-75% of their patients were 7th to 9th graders; the remaining 4% indicated that 76-100% of their patients were 7th to 9th graders.

Forty-four percent of SAM respondents were involved in organized health education programs for adolescents at the time of their participation in the study. These programs were school-based (40%), community-based (28%), medical facility-based (16%), and a combination of these (16%).

American School Health Association. The 338 respondents represented 34% of the sample of 986 from ASHA who received the survey. Three hundred twenty-nine of these had complete data and could be analyzed. Further description of results will refer to these respondents.

Nineteen percent of ASHA respondents were male, 81% were female. Fifty-three percent of respondents were 30-49 years old; an additional 26% were 40-49. Fifty-three percent were nurses, and 33% were health educators. Of the remaining number, 5% specified training in general education, and 6% specified areas including medicine, public health, social work, and psychology. Location of work was largely urban (42%), followed closely by suburban (35%) and rural (23%). The amount of their work targeted at 7th to 9th graders varied, with 40% having 1-25% of their work targeted at this age group, 18% having 26-50% of their work focus on 7th to 9th graders; and 9% focusing 51-75% of their work on this age group.

Fifty-six percent of the respondents were involved in organized health education programs for adolescents at the time of their response. An overwhelming majority of these, 89%, were school-based.

Importance Ratings

Table 1 presents the frequency of respondents' rating each health issue as "very important." Chi square analysis revealed differences between SAM and ASHA members for how important it is for students to learn to eat healthy food ($x^2 1=53.3$, $p<.0001$), to learn to handle pressures to engage in sexual intercourse ($x^2 1=14.4$, $p<.0001$), and to learn to handle pressures to use the drug marijuana ($x^2 1=12.3$, $p<.0001$). Members of ASHA were more likely to perceive these issues as very important.

Multidimensional Scaling Dimensions

For both organizations, the arrangement of points was virtually identical for the split halves of data. The stress levels of the data on the SAM data were .236 and .230, and on the ASHA data were .243 and .233. These stress values were consistent, and moderately good, thereby establishing a multidimensional solution to the similarity data (Young and Lewyckyj, 1981). The variance accounted for by the solution ranged from .661 and .671 for the SAM data to .676 and .703 for the ASHA data. These are, again, reasonably good amounts of variance to be accounted for by the multidimensional configuration (Young and Lewyckyj, 1981).

The configuration which results from the MDS analysis of the data from both groups (see Figure 1) shows the nine health issues arranged along two dimensions and in groups in multidimensional space. The first step in interpreting the dimensions was to look at the characteristics of the health issues at each end of a dimension to determine if there was some attribute that distinguished them in an obvious way (Schiffman et al., 1981). Table 2 lists the order of health issues along each of the two dimensions.

Dimension 1. For SAM members, Dimension 1, the horizontal dimension, had an overall importance rating of .4903; for ASHA members, it had an importance rating of .4501. The health issues at opposite ends of this dimension were failing to care for skin properly, and the use of drugs such as amphetamines, barbiturates, and hallucinogens. These two health issues differ in terms of the seriousness of the health consequences of the two behaviors. An examination of the health issues along the continuum between these two health issues supports an interpretation of this dimension as depicting perceived seriousness of health consequences.

Dimension 2. For SAM members, Dimension 2, the vertical dimension, had an overall importance rating of .1757; for ASHA members, it had an importance rating of .2394. The health issues at opposite ends of Dimension 2 are smoking cigarettes, and engaging in sexual intercourse. The interpretation of the arrangement of issues along this dimension is more ambiguous. This arrangement may reflect the respondents' perceptions of the susceptibility of 7th to 9th graders to the issues, or it may reflect the extent to which implications of the risk are perceived as immediate vs. long term.

Grouping of Issues in Multidimensional Space. The arrangement of the nine health issues was also interpreted in terms of the groups they formed in multidimensional space. The configuration suggested that the issues formed groups by subject matter (see Table 3). Skin care and nutrition were independent of each other and of the other health concerns. Cigarettes, marijuana, inhalants, and drugs such as amphetamines, barbiturates, and hallucinogens formed a group which was named Substance Abuse Issues. Sexual intercourse, child abuse, and drunk driving formed a group which was named Socially Oriented Health Concerns.

Importance Ratings and Multidimensional Scaling Configurations

The importance ratings and the MDS dimensions and groupings were examined to assess the extent to which perceived similarity among issues provided a basis for determining the importance of health issues for inclusion in health promotion programs targeted at young teens. The importance ratings of the health issues are in general agreement with their arrangement along Dimension 1, with the exception of the issues of sexual intercourse and child abuse. Drunk driving and drugs and nutrition and skin care anchor opposite ends of both displays. There was no apparent correspondence between the arrangement of health issues along Dimension 2 and the importance ratings of the same health issues.

DISCUSSION

A traditional approach to the interpretation of importance or priority ratings might include the correlation of measures of importance of the issues and measures of suspected bases for importance ratings (e.g., severity, susceptibility, experience with the issue). Another approach to this study might include the regression of perceived importance and other attributes of a health issue on a measure of intention to conduct programs related to the health issue. Both approaches would be looking for linear relationships. The present study measured importance and allowed other dimensions to emerge. This approach expected and allowed for the multidimensional nature of reflection regarding health issues by health professionals. While this approach produced results that reflect similarity rather than the expected differences in the underlying perceptions of the two groups of respondents, the presence of similarity in perception adds information rather than acts as an end point to this line of research.

School Health and Adolescent Medicine respondents had many areas of agreement regarding appropriate areas for intervention to protect the health and well being of 7th to 9th graders. Significant differences were noted in only three areas. ASHA respondents were more likely than SAM respondents to emphasize nutrition, sexual intercourse, and marijuana. Areas of agreement may best be stressed in cooperative efforts to develop health promotion programs since both groups represent professionals whose care is vital to the young teen.

More usually applied in assessing preferences for products in marketing efforts, MDS was used in the present study to measure respondents' cognitive appraisal of health issues. The resulting spatial display has stimulated discussion of the meaning of the placement of health issues along two dimensions of the display, and of the grouping of certain of the nine health issues. Additional semantic evaluation of the issues would allow more direct interpretation of their placement. For example, randomly selected respondents within a total sample could be asked to complete questionnaires which would allow MDS analysis. Other randomly selected segments of the sample could be asked to complete semantic scales of the issues using suspected interpretations of the dimensions revealed by analysis of the MDS data (e.g., salience to target group, severity of consequences, degree of control over exposure to the issue). Agreement between placement along dimensions and one or more semantic scales would indicate areas of potential intervention to influence the selection process.

It was anticipated that the physicians who were members of SAM were primarily, if not exclusively, involved in direct health care delivery, and that members of ASHA were predominantly involved in educational efforts in school settings. From this difference in the settings in which physicians, school nurses, and health educators apply their training, as well as from the health or illness-related circumstances under which the two groups encounter teens (Levenson et al., 1984), it was expected that the professional societies, which are composed primarily of these different professional groups, would differ in their perceptions of the issues.

Such differences have previously been identified (Levenson et al., 1986). However, 44% of SAM respondents reported being involved in health education programs for adolescents at the time of their participation in the study. Of these, 40% were school-based, and an additional 16% were a combination of school- and community-based programs. This corresponds to the members of ASHA, 56% of whom were involved in adolescent health education programs, 89% of which were school-based. This shared programmatic involvement, even though through different professional roles, is likely to have a major impact on shaping perceptions. A review of Table 1 reveals that respondents from both groups rated almost all nine issues as very important for inclusion. While this congruency of perspective is programmatically encouraging, this concordance on importance might indicate that there may not have been, after all, sufficient variation in respondents' perceptions of the importance of the issues for differences to be validly indicated by the MDS analysis. With greater variation of importance ratings, the spatial display might account for greater variance and decrease the stress level in the data, thus allowing clearer interpretation of meanings of the arrangement of health issues to respondents.

The MDS data (Figure 1) indicate that issues are perceived in cognitive groups of related general concerns rather than in linear arrangements of individual items. This includes a group of substance abuse issues which included drugs such as amphetamines, barbiturates, hallucinogens; cigarettes; inhalants; and marijuana, and a group of social health concerns which included drunk driving, sexual intercourse for this age group, and child abuse (see Table 3). The similar grouping of concerns suggests that these health professionals view certain health issues as sharing common components. With the present emphasis on a comprehensive approach to both health education and care for adolescents, these results are compatible with the importance of broad-based approaches to health education planning rather than a narrow, item specific focus.

These professional organizations are on the front line of health promotion initiatives. The groups share priorities and concerns which might be mobilized effectively on national, state, and local levels to influence decisions regarding community health education policy and programming. The extent to which the strong public health focus of the members of SAM and ASHA is representative of adolescent medicine pediatricians and family practice physicians, or school nurses and health educators, nationally is not known. Subsequent studies might address this. If these organizations do distinguish themselves in this regard, they might be highly effective in informing other members of the health community of the need and opportunities in practice for comprehensive community based responses which address maladaptive behavioral practices of adolescents. In the present paper, the authors seek to demonstrate how the utilization of Multidimensional Scaling may serve to provide some additional perspective on responses from these groups concerning their perceived health priorities for adolescents.

Project supported as a component of "Bio-behavioral Collaboration in Adolescent Health Promotion" Grant #MCJ-483288, Division of Maternal and Child Health, Bureau of Health Care Delivery and Assistance, U.S. Department of Health and Human Services.

REFERENCES

Ajzen, I. & Fishbein, M. (1973). Attitudinal and normative variables as predictors of specific behaviors. *Journal of Personality and Social Psychology, 27(1)*, 41-57.

Alba, J.W. & Hasher, L. (1983). Is memory schematic? *Psychological Bulletin, 93(2)*, 203-231.

Blum, R. & Smith, M. (1988). Training of health professionals in adolescent health care: Study group report. *Journal of Adolescent Health Care, 9 (6 supplement)*, 465-505.

Dratt, L.M. (1985). The effects of question format and group membership on the selection of factors important to the health of adolescents (Masters thesis, University of Houston, 1984). *Masters Abstracts International.*

Dratt, L.M. & Evans, R.I. (1985). *Social communication feedback loop and prevention program focus selection.* Unpublished manuscript.

Fortenberry, J.D., Kaplan, D.W., & Hill, R.F. (1988). Physicians' values and experience during adolescence: Their effect on adolescent health care. *Journal of Adolescent Health Care, 9,* 46-51.

Hochbaum, G. (1958). Public participation in medical screening programs: A socio-psychological study (PHS Publication No. 572). Washington, D.C.: U.S. Government Printing Office.

Iverson, D.C. & Kolbe, L.J. (1983). Evolution of the national disease prevention and health promotion strategy: Establishing a role for the schools. *Journal of School Health, 53,* 294-302.

Kruskal, J.B. & Wish, M. (1978). Basic concepts of multidimensional scaling. *Multidimensional Scaling.* Beverly Hills: Sage Publications.

Levenson, P.M., Morrow, J.R., Johnson, S.A., & Pfefferbaum, B.J. (1984). Assessing adolescent health needs: A factor analytic approach. *Patient Education and Counseling, 5,* 23-29.

Levenson, P.M., Morrow, J.R., Morgan, W.C., & Pfefferbaum, B.J. (1985). Health information sources and preferences as perceived by adolescents, pediatricians, teachers, and school nurses. *Journal of Early Adolescence, 6(2),* 183-196.

Nisbett, R.E. & Wilson, T.D. (1977). Telling more than we can know: Verbal reports on mental processes. *Psychological Review, 84(3)*, 231-259.

Parcel, G.S., Nader, P.R., & Meyer, M.P. (1977). Adolescent health concerns, problems, and patterns of utilization in a triethnic urban population. *Pediatrics, 6*, 157-164.

Rosenstock, I.M. (1974). Historical origins of the health belief model. In M.H. Becker (Ed.) The health belief model and personal health behavior. *Health Education Monographs, 2(4)*, 328-335.

Schiffman, S.S., Reynolds, M.L. & Young, F.W. (1981). *Introduction to multidimensional scaling.* New York: Academic Press, Inc.

Smith, J.K., Falvo, D., McKillip, J., & Pitz, G. (1984). Measuring patient perceptions of the patient-doctor interaction. *Evaluation and the Health Professions, 7(1)*, 77-94.

Subkoviak, M.J. (1975). The use of multidimensional scaling in educational research. *Review of Educational Research, 45(3)*, 387-423.

Tversky, A. & Kahneman, D. (September, 1974). Judgment under uncertainty: Heuristics and biases. *Science, 185*, 1124-1131.

Young, F.W. & Lewyckyj, R. (1981). *Alscal-4 user's guide* (2nd ed.). Chapel Hill, N.C.: Institutes for Research in the Social Sciences, UNC.

Table 1. Distribution by Group Membership of Respondents' Choice of "Very Important" by Health Issue

	Group Membership					
	SAM (n=451)			ASHA (n=329)		
Health Issue	Order	n	%	Order	n	%
Drunk Driving	1	359	81	2	266	81
Drugs	2	347	78	2	266	81
Sexual Intercourse [a]	3	324	73	1	273	83
Cigarettes	4	314	71	5	242	74
Inhalants	5	299	67	6	224	68
Marijuana [a]	6	295	67	4	252	77
Child Abuse	7	268	60	8	188	57
Nutrition [a]	8	180	41	7	216	66
Skin Care	9	63	14	9	61	17

[a] $p < .0001$

Table 2. Arrangement of Health Issues across Dimensions 1 and 2 for both SAM and ASHA

Dimension 1	Dimension 2
Drugs	Cigarettes
Drunk driving	Marijuana
Child abuse	Inhalants
Inhalants	Drugs
Marijuana	Nutrition
Cigarettes	Skin care
Sexual intercourse	Drunk driving
Nutrition	Child abuse
Skin care	Sexual intercourse

Table 3. Grouping of Health Issues in Multidimensional Space

Social Concerns	Substance Abuse	Diet	Hygiene
Drunk Driving	Drugs	Nutrition	Skin Care
Sexual Intercourse	Cigarettes		
Child Abuse	Inhalants		
	Marijuana		

Figure 1. Configuration representing similarity data on health issues "in terms of long-term health consequences" for 7-9th graders in general (n=780).

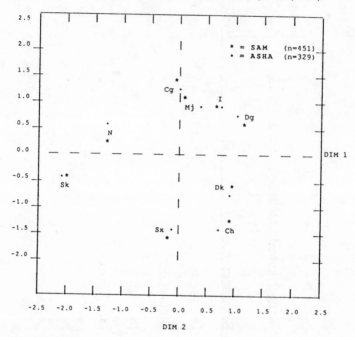

Health Issue Legend
Dk = Riding with drivers who are or have been drinking
Dg = Using drugs such as amphetamines, barbiturates, hallucinogens
Sx = Engaging in sexual intercourse
Cg = Smoking cigarettes
I   = Sniffing paint, glue, or other substances
Mj = Using the drug marijuana
Ch = Failing to report or get help for child abuse
N   = Having unhealthy eating habits
Sk = Failing to care for skin properly

8

THE RELATIONSHIP OF INTERNAL AND EXTERNAL MOTIVATIONAL FACTORS TO EXERCISE AND DIETARY HABITS OF COLLEGE STUDENTS

Lillian Cook Carter
Walter Greene

This study was designed to identify those persons with good exercise and dietary habits and those with poor exercise and dietary habits in order to compare these groups with respect to the following: their attitudes toward physical activity and nutrition; their self motivation; and family influences on physical activity and nutrition. A secondary purpose was to determine the ability of these variables to predict exercise and dietary habits.

A sample of 278 college students completed a physical activities diary (PAD), a dietary recall (DR), Petrie's Attitude Toward Physical Activities survey, Sim's Attitude Toward Nutrition survey, Dishman's Self Motivation Inventory, and a questionnaire on family influences. The results of the PAD and DR indicated that 66% had poor exercise habits and 68% has poor dietary habits. A significant difference (p<.01) in attitudes toward physical activity was found between subjects with good and poor exercise habits; those with good exercise habits reporting more positive attitudes. In addition, there was a significant difference (p<.05) found between overweight and underweight subjects with respect to their attitudes toward physical activity; underweight subjects showed a more positive attitude. Attitudes toward nutrition and subjects' self-motivation were found to be unrelated to exercise or dietary habits. An inverse relationship was found between the amount of encouragement given to the subject

175

father and mother to exercise and eat nutritiously, and the subject's exercise and dietary habits. The ability to classify subjects into the correct exercise and dietary groups through use of the selected predictors was limited.

The resurgence of public interest in physical fitness and nutrition has been welcomed by most health educators. The health impact of habitual participation in vigorous exercise and the benefits of eating nutritiously are both well established. Among the many benefits is the recent finding that adequate exercise over a lifetime can add one to two years of additional life by the age of eighty (Pattenbarger et al., 1986). It is also speculated that improved nutrition may decrease the illness and morbidity associated with aging (Sandstead, 1985).

The contention that good exercise habits in combination with good dietary habits can contribute significantly to improving the health of an individual is relatively easy to establish. More difficult, however, is the task of determining the *factors* that will elicit this sort of behavior. Clearly, the mere possession of the knowledge that a certain behavior will improve the quality of life does not necessarily cause a person to adopt favorable health behaviors (Henderson et al., 1979).

In an attempt to identify the factors that differentiate those who exercise and eat nutritiously from those with poor exercise and dietary habits, the investigators examined the attitudes toward physical activity and nutrition, the self motivation and the influences of the family on exercise and dietary habits.

Attitudes, according to Sherif and Sherif (1969, p. 334), "are inferred from characteristic, consistent and selective modes of behavior directed toward or against relevant objects and events." Attitudes help to motivate and contribute to making a behavior routine (Carruth & Anderson, 1977). Rosenstock (1960) views all behavior as a function of a person's motives and his or her beliefs about various opportunities for action. The support given by a person's family to continue a behavior has also been identified as an influencing factor (Heinzelman & Bagley, 1970; Carruth et al., 1977; Andrew & Parker, 1979; Foss, 1980). With these considerations in mind, this study was designed to identify those persons with good exercise and dietary habits. These groups were compared with respect to their attitudes toward physical activity and nutrition, as well as their self-motivation and family influences on physical activity and nutrition. A secondary purpose of the study was to determine the ability of these variables to predict exercise and dietary behavior.

METHODOLOGY

Sample Selection

The study involved a representative group of college students enrolled in an elective, general health education course. These subjects were volunteers from 8 sections randomly selected from 16 sections taught that semester. Of 285 possible participants, 283 volunteered to participate. Five of these failed to complete the instrument and were eliminated as subjects, thus leaving 278 participants.

Data Collection

All data was collected from each of the eight sections during the seventy-five minute scheduled class period. The assessments were made prior to the time that the topics of exercise and nutrition were scheduled for discussion.

Instruments

Exercise Habits. Exercise habits were assessed with a physical activities survey, measuring the subjects' most vigorous 30 minutes of activity for the previous 7 days. These types of surveys have been widely used, are easy to administer and seem to provide reliable results (Yasin et al., 1967; Buskirk et al., 1971; Taylor et al., 1978; Thacker, 1981). The recall instrument used in this study was employed by Thacker (1981) in validating the Canadian Home Fitness Test. Thacker (1981) found strong correlations between fitness levels and the most intense 15 minutes of activity per day. In the present study those who engaged in strenuous activity (level

260 - 1255 for 30 minutes three times per week or level 260 -
1255 two times per week and level 180 - 230 two times per week)
were categorized as having good exercise habits. Some examples
of the activities and corresponding levels are: walking a 15-minute
mile=level 180; competitive singles tennis=level 310; jogging an
11-minute mile=level 355; field or ice hockey=level 460. Those
not achieving these levels were categorized as having poor exercise
habits. This standard is used by Foss (1980) and is taken from the
position statement of the American College of Sports Medicine on
the quality and quantity of exercise.

Dietary Habits. A twenty-four hour dietary recall was used
to assess the nutritional intake of each student. Twenty-four hour
dietary recalls are a major tool used in assessing food intake.

In their review of the literature, Stunkard and Waxman
(1981) found self report of food intake to be relatively accurate.
They recommended that twenty-four hour recalls be regarded with
greater confidence than they were then accorded. This opinion is
supported by Pao, Mickel and Burk (1985) who examined 8,779
nutrient intakes of individuals participating in the Spring of 1977
Nationwide Food Consumption Survey.

In the present study, the dietary recalls were tabulated using
a dietary score of 0-16 based on a system devised by Guthrie and
Scheer (1981). This scoring system is based on the assumption
that diets providing foods from the four major food groups can
provide the foundation for an adequate intake and that each food
group has a unique nutritional make up that contributes to dietary
adequacy. Those subjects scoring 13 to 16 points and not omitting
any food group were placed in the good dietary habits group, and
all other subjects were placed in the poor dietary habits group. A
measure of energy balance was used as an additional check on the
validity of the measures of exercise and dietary habits. Each
subject's height and weight was measured and compared to the
Metropolitan Life Insurance Tables (1959). Subjects classified as
having both good exercise and dietary habits yet measuring 10%
overweight would have been eliminated from the study since their
weight appears to contradict the exercise and dietary habits group
placement. However, no subjects required elimination based on
this criterion.

Attitudes Toward Physical Activity and Nutrition. Attitude toward physical activity was assessed using a modification of Kenyon's Attitude Toward Physical Activity survey developed by Petrie (1971a; 1971b). This ten-question survey is answered on a seven-point scale ranging from very strongly disagree to very strongly agree. The survey statements address the degree of support a subject expresses for various motivations for physical activity. Attitude toward nutrition was assessed with a scale which was devised by Eppright (1970) and shortened by Sims (1978). The scale is divided into three sections: nutrition is important; meal planning is important; meal preparation is enjoyable. Answers ranged along a five-point Likert type scale from strongly agree to strongly disagree.

Self Motivation and Family Influences. Self motivation, described by Dishman as a nonspecific tendency to persist in habitual behavior regardless of extrinsic reinforcement, was measured using an inventory devised by Dishman and Ickes (1981). The amount of encouragement given subjects by their family members to be physically active and to have good dietary habits was assessed using an investigator designed 8-item questionnaire with a Likert-type scale. Subjects responded to the following statements using a 5-point range from strongly agree to strongly disagree: (1) from as early as I can remember while growing up, the following people encouraged me to be physically active and/or participate in sports; (2) from as early as I can remember while growing up, the following people encouraged me to eat nutritious, "good for me" foods. The family members listed included father, mother, brother(s), and sister(s).

RESULTS

Exercise and Dietary Habits

The majority of the respondents were classified as having poor exercise habits (66%) and poor dietary habits (68%) based on the physical activities diary and dietary recall. Only 13% of the sample could be classified as having both good exercise and good dietary habits. Of this group, 72% were male. Subjects classified as having both poor exercise and poor dietary habits comprised a much larger group (45% of the respondents) with 66% of this group being female.

The comparison of each subject's height and weight to the 1959 Metropolitan Life Insurance Tables determined that 18% of the respondents were 10% or more over ideal body weight for height. Seven percent of the sample proved to be underweight for their height by 10% or greater. The overweight subjects ranged as high as 80% over ideal body weight while the underweight subjects ranged only as high as 20% below ideal body weight.

Attitudes Toward Physical Activity

The analysis of variance revealed a significant difference (p<.01) between the good exercise habits group and the poor exercise habits group with respect to their attitudes toward physical activity. Those in the good exercise habits group indicated more positive attitudes toward physical activity with male subjects showing significantly more positive (p<.01) attitudes than females. An analysis of variance was also performed to compare the attitudes toward physical activity of those in the three weight categories: ideal, overweight, and underweight. A significant difference (p<.05) was found between the attitudes of the subjects in the two extreme weight categories. The underweight subjects indicated the most positive attitudes toward physical activity with the overweight subjects expressing the least support for physical activity.

Attitudes Toward Nutrition

The analysis of variance did not reveal any significant difference between those subjects in the good dietary habits group and those in the poor dietary habits group with respect to their attitudes toward nutrition. However, as shown in Table 1, the analysis of variance revealed that the males indicated a significantly more positive response than females (p<.05) in the category "meal preparation is important." Table 2 illustrates a significant two-way interaction which was found between attitude toward nutrition, nutrition category, and weight. The highest score (i.e., indicating the most positive attitude toward nutrition) was reported in those underweight subjects in the good dietary habits group. The lowest mean attitude score was also reported in the underweight category but by those in the poor dietary group (p<.02).

Self Motivation

Males were found to have significantly higher (p<.05) levels of self-motivation than females based on Dishman's Self-Motivation Inventory. No significant differences in self-motivation between the good and poor exercise, and the good and poor dietary habits groups were found.

Family Influences

Sixty-three percent of the sample reported receiving encouragement from their fathers to be physically active and 57% reported being encouraged by their mothers. A high level of encouragement to eat nutritious food was also reported. Sixty-nine percent of the sample received encouragement from their fathers to eat nutritiously, while 90% received similar encouragement from their mothers. Figure 3 illustrates the inverse relationship between encouragement to eat nutritiously and active dietary habits. A significantly higher (p<.05) amount of encouragement to eat nutritiously was given by the family of those subjects in the poor dietary habits group compared to those subjects in the good dietary habits group. This trend was also found in encouragement given by father and mother where those in the poor dietary habits group again received more encouragement (p<.05) to eat well (data not shown). In both exercise and dietary habits groups, those with good habits reported receiving less encouragement from their fathers and mothers than those with poor habits. These differences were significant at the 0.06 level for exercise and the 0.05 level for dietary habits.

When weight categories were compared with respect to nutritional encouragement, a significant difference (p<.05) was found between underweight and overweight subjects; the underweight subjects indicated receiving the most encouragement to eat nutritiously while the overweight subjects received the least encouragement.

Ability of Variables to Predict Group Membership

A stepwise multiple discriminant function analysis was used to determine if the independent variables of this study could be used to predict group membership (Huck et al., 1974). Specifically, this analysis was performed to determine if exercise and dietary habits could be predicted based on attitude toward physical activity, attitude toward nutrition, self-motivation, and family influences. This effort met with only minimal success. The predictor variables were only able to correctly classify 58% of the subjects into the correct exercise group and 58% into the correct dietary group. Since 50% could be correctly classified by chance, these percentages were judged to be too low for use as predictors by exercise and dietary habits.

DISCUSSION

Exercise and Dietary Habits

The findings of this study indicate that the majority of this sample (66%) had poor exercise habits. Although we appear to be in an era of fitness consciousness, the majority of the general population seems not to participate in vigorous routine physical activity. A recent study of 16,936 Harvard Alumni classified 62% of the sample as sedentary, a finding similar to the present study (Pattenbarger, 1986). The majority of the present sample (68%) also appeared to have poor dietary habits. This finding is similar to those of a recent survey of the eating habits of 421 college students. A 24-hour dietary assessment showed 75% of those subjects as having "fair" or "poor" intakes (Marrale et al., 1986).

Attitudes Toward Physical Activity

Those subjects with good exercise habits had more positive attitudes toward physical activity. The males showed more involvement in physical activity and the attitudes toward physical activity scores of the males were significantly higher than the scores of the females. These findings support the findings of Kenyon (1968) whose study indicated that attitudes were directly related to primary and secondary involvement in physical activity.

Attitudes Toward Nutrition

The variable of attitude toward nutrition did not distinguish between those with good and those with poor dietary habits. Surprisingly, this survey has been used previously by Eppright (1970) and Swartz (1975) showing significant correlations between attitude and practice.

Eppright (1970) showed that mothers of children with the lowest nutrient intakes tended to have the least favorable attitudes toward meal planning, food preparation, and nutrition. The scores showed a similar trend in the present study in two of the three categories. Those subjects with poor dietary habits had lower mean scores in the two attitude categories "nutrition is important" and "meal planning is important" than did those in the good category; however, the differences were not significant.

In support of the attitude findings of this study are the findings of Perron and Endress (1985) who found attitude toward nutrition was not a good predictor of dietary behavior. These authors had attempted to determine the relationship between nutrition knowledge, attitude, and dietary practices of 27 female adolescent athletes.

Self-Motivation

The self-motivation data of the current study yielded results which differed from those found in the literature. Dishman and

Ickes (1981) were able to correctly classify 80% of a sample of therapeutic exercise subjects into dropouts and adherers in a discriminant analysis using the variables percent body fat, self-motivation, and weight. In the present study self-motivation did not contribute to correct classification of subjects. It is possible that the samples used by Dishman were not representative of the general population. His first sample consisted of female athletes and the second of volunteers in a therapeutic exercise program. These two groups may be more highly motivated than the general population. This could be one explanation for the difference in the mean scores for Dishman's studies and the present study.

Family Influences

It appears that much encouragement was given to subjects by both father and mother to exercise and eat nutritiously. Somewhat surprising, however, was a trend of more parental encouragement in the groups that did not exercise or eat nutritiously. Reliability and validity coefficients need to be determined for this instrument before speculating on the cause of these results.

Combined Grouping

When those subjects who were classified as having both good exercise and good dietary habits were compared to those subjects having both poor exercise and poor dietary habits, body weight proved to be the strongest predictor of group membership. It is possible that the weight of the subjects is an outward manifestation of his or her exercise and dietary habits. In contrast, the information gathered using paper and pencil for the other variables may have been manipulated and slanted toward what the subjects wished to portray while weight showed actual behavior.

CONCLUSIONS

Based upon the information showing such a high percentage of either poor exercise habits, poor dietary habits, or both poor exercise and dietary habits among college students, it is obvious that more emphasis needs to be placed on education in the area of exercise and nutrition. Further research is needed to determine motivators for these health promoting behaviors so that education in these areas can produce positive, lifelong behavior changes.

REFERENCES

Andrew, G. & Parker, J. (1979). Factors related to dropout of post myocardial infarction patients from exercise programs. *Medicine and Science in Sports, 11,* 376-378.

Buskirk, E., Harris, D., Mendez, J. & Skinner, J. (1971). Comparison of two assessments of physical activity and a survey of methods for caloric intake. *The American Journal of Clinical Nutrition, 24,* 1119-1125.

Carruth, B. & Anderson, H. (1977). Scaling criteria in developing and evaluating an attitude instrument. *Journal of the American Dietetic Association, 73,* 42-47.

Carruth, B., Mangel, M. & Anderson, H. (1977). Assessing change-proneness and nutrition related behaviors. *Journal of the American Dietetic Association, 70,* 47-53.

Dishman, R. & Ickes, W. (1981). Self motivation and adherence to therapeutic exercise. *Journal of Behavioral Medicine, 4,* 421-438.

Eppright, E., Fox, M., Fryer, B., Lamken, G. & Vivian, V. (1970). Nutrition knowledge and attitudes of mothers. *Journal of Home Economics, 62,* 327-332.

Foss, P. (1980). Brief reports: Physical activity and attitudes surveyed. *The Physician and Sports Medicine, 8,* 22.

Guthrie, H. & Scheer, J. (1981). Validity of a dietary score for assessing nutrient adequacy. *Journal of the American Dietetic Association, 78,* 240-244.

Heinzelman, F. & Bagley, R. (1970). Response to physical activity programs and their effects on health behaviors. *Public Health Reports, 7,* 366-373.

Henderson, J., Hall, S. & Lipton, H. (1979). Changing self-destructive behaviors. In C. Stone et al. (Eds.) *Health Psychology.* San Francisco: Jossey-Bass.

Kenyon, G. (1968). *Values held for physical activity by selected urban secondary school students in Canada, Australia, England and the United States.* Washington, D.C.: United States Office of Education.

Marrale, J., Shipman, J. & Rhodes, M. (1968). What some college students eat. *Nutrition Today,* Jan-Feb, 16-21.

Metropolitan Life Insurance Company (1959). *How to control your weight,* New York.

Pao, E., Meckle, S. & Burk, M. (1981). One-day and 3-day nutrient intakes by individuals: Nationwide food consumption survey findings, spring 1977. *Journal of the American Dietetic Association, 85,* 3, 313-324.

Pattenbarger, R., Hyde, R., Wing, A. & Hsieh, C. (1986). Physical activity, all-cause mortality and longevity of college alumni. *The New England Journal of Medicine, 314,* 10, 605-613.

Petrie, B. (1971a). Achievement orientations in adolescent attitudes towards play. *International Review of Sports Sociology, 6,* 81-99.

Petrie, B. (1971b). Achievement orientations in the motivations of Canadian University students towards physical activity. *Journal of the Canadian Association of Health, Physical Education, and Recreation, 37,* 7-13.

Rosenstock, I. (1960). What research in motivation suggests for public health. *American Journal Public Health, 3,* 295-302.

Sandstead, H. (1985). Some relationships between nutrition and aging. *Journal of the American Dietetic Association, 85,* 2, 171-173.

Sims, L. (1978). Dietary status of lactating women. *Journal of the American Dietetic Association, 73,* 147-154.

Stunkard, A. & Waxman, M. (1981). Accuracy of self-reports of food intake. *Journal of the American Dietetic Association, 79,* 547-551.

Swartz, N. (1975). Nutrition knowledge, attitudes, and practices of high school graduates. *Journal of the American Dietetic Association, 66,* 28-31.

Taylor, H., Jacobs, D., Schucker, B., Knudsen, J., Leon, A., & Debacker, G. (1978). A questionnaire for the assessment of leisure time physical activities. *Journal of Chronic Diseases, 31,* 741-755.

Thacker, J. (1981). The validation of selected physical activity questions using the Canadian home fitness test. *Canadian Journal of Public Health, 72,* 455-458.

Yasin, S., Alderson, M., Marr, J., Pattison, D. & Morris, J. (1967). Assessment of habitual physical activity apart from occupation. *British Journal of Preventive Social Medicine, 21,* 163-169.

Table 1

MEAN SCORES ON ATTITUDE TOWARD NUTRITION

	MALES	FEMALES	POSSIBLE RANGE[a]
Nutrition is important	18.12	17.99	6-30
Meal planning is important	15.26	15.27	6-30
Meal preparation is important	20.88	10.01*	7-35
Total mean score	54.51	53.36	19-95

[a]Higher score indicates more positive attitude.

* p <.05

Table 2

RESULTS OF A DUNCAN MULTIPLE COMPARISON TEST OF ATTITUDES
TOWARD NUTRITION REPORTED BY THE UNDERLINING METHOD[a]

Nutrition Category	Ideal Weight	Overweight	Underweight
Good	53.22	55.17	59.67
Poor	54.46	53.08	51.83*

[a]Comparison of mean attitudes toward nutrition made within good and poor nutrition category with respect to 3 weight groups and between good and poor nutrition category within each weight group.

*A significant difference (p <.02) was found in attitudes among underweight subjects in the good and poor nutrition category.

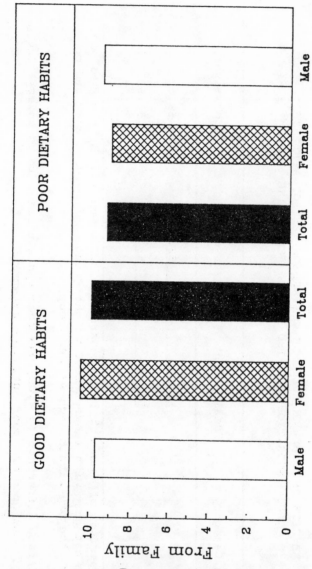

9

THE EFFECT OF PHYSICAL ACTIVITY ON SELF-ASSESSED LIFE SATISFACTION AND HEALTH STATUS IN THE ELDERLY

Catherine A. Kennedy
Sandra M. Schleiffers

One hundred and fifty uninstitutionalized men and women 60 years of age and older participated in this study which was conducted to examine the effect of physical activity on self-assessed life satisfaction and health status. All subjects were selected on the basis of a personal rating of fair for these parameters. Subjects were randomly assigned to either walking or control conditions. Further, subjects assigned to the walking condition were randomly assigned to either walk-alone or walk-in-pairs groups. Control group subjects continued normal activities throughout the study, while subjects assigned to the walking groups were required to walk 4 x 45 min/week for a 15-week period. Following the 15-week period, life satisfaction and health status were re-assessed. Two 2 x 3 ANOVAs demonstrated a significant difference among the group conditions for both life satisfaction and health status ($F=80.28$, $F=57.71$, [$p<.05$] respectively). Subsequently, post hoc analyses demonstrated a significant difference between the walking condition groups and the control group ($p<.05$). These results lend support to existing reports of improved self-perception following participation in physical activity.

While concern for adaptation to aging has flourished, more interest is being paid to the concept of life satisfaction or dissatisfaction of elderly persons (Edwards & Klemmack, 1973; Kennedy et al.,

1983; Markides & Martin, 1979; Neugarten et al., 1961; Palmore & Kivett, 1977; Spreitzer & Snyder, 1974). Of the many variables studied, self-assessed health status has repeatedly proven to be a significant predictor of life satisfaction (Edwards & Klemmack, 1973; Hansen & Yoshioka, 1963; Kennedy et al., 1983; Mancini, 1981; Sonquist et al., 1973; Spreitzer & Larson, 1979). It is assumed that physical activity not only influences life satisfaction but also plays a major role in health status which in turn impacts on life satisfaction (de Vries, 1974).

Presently, there exists a concentrated effort on the part of many sources to improve the level of physical activity among a variety of populations. Much of the scholarly work performed in this area centralizes on the impact of physical activity on younger individuals. Research involving the aging adult has concentrated on improved physical functioning in controlled training programs (Ray et al., 1983). Although these investigations have demonstrated positive results in the physiological literature, there has been a paucity of research documenting increased health status and life satisfaction as a result of physical activity. Therefore, whether elderly participation in physical activity has a positive influence on life satisfaction or not is for the moment largely supposition (de Vries, 1974; Hammett, 1967). A possible explanation for this is the numerous methodologies that have been employed causing a lack of uniformity and consensus. For example, procedural diversities have included: (a) method of exercise employed, (b) type of exercise program, and (c) measurements utilized to define psychological functioning (Benestad, 1965; Gutman et al., 1977; Ray et al., 1983; Sidney & Shephard, 1977; Stamford et al., 1974).

Much of the research involving elderly participation in physical activity has focused on the atypical population (Blue, 1979; Harris & Frankel, 1977; Kavanaugh et al., 1973; Powell, 1974). Few investigations reported in the literature have involved uninstitutionalized and independently functioning older adults. However, these few studies have resulted in findings supportive of improved self esteem, alteration of mood and personality, and disposition (Hanson & Nedde, 1974; Massie & Shephard, 1971; Ray et al., 1983). Therefore, the purpose of this study was to investigate the effect of a 15-week walking program on self-assessed life satisfaction and health status of independently functioning adults 60 years of age and older.

METHODS AND PROCEDURES

Instrumentation

The questionnaire utilized to evaluate self-assessed life satisfaction and health status was developed by King & Muraco (1980). This instrument consists of selected items utilized as multiple predictors of these parameters. Subjects respond to the items on the questionnaire based on a scale ranging from poor (poor=1) to excellent (excellent=4).

Subjects

Subjects were selected from a larger pool consisting of 900 residents, 60 years of age or older, residing in Fort Collins, Colorado. A sample of 226 subjects was singled out on the basis of subject responses on the questionnaire of fair (fair=2) for both life satisfaction and health status.

Each of the selected subjects was contacted by phone to: (a) request participation in the study, and (b) explain the study. Of the 226 subjects, 150 agreed to participate in the study.

Subjects were randomly assigned to a control group ($\underline{n}$=50), a walking-alone group ($\underline{n}$=50), and a walking-in-pairs group ($\underline{n}$=50). Proof of a physical examination within 6 months prior to the experiment and completion of a Health Risk Appraisal were required of all subjects assigned to the walking conditions. Further, a letter was sent to each subject's physician which explained the experiment and requested a statement from the physician regarding approval of subject participation. The physician was asked to respond with an over-all evaluation of the subject's health. Of the 150 subjects who agreed to participate in the study, five did not complete the walking program. Specifically, two subjects assigned to the walking-in-pairs group and three subjects assigned to the walking-alone group did not complete the study.

Implementation

Prior to implementing the walking program, an initial group meeting was organized to describe the study in detail. Each subject was asked to walk 4 x 45 min/week for a period of 15 weeks with no stipulation concerning distance walked or pace. Although distance walked was not a factor in this study, each subject assigned to a walking group was supplied with a pedometer and asked to keep track of distance traveled for each walking session. This was instituted as a control to ensure that the subjects actually walked according to schedule. Handouts concerning attire, suitable times to walk, and warm-up and cool-down techniques were given to each subject and explained thoroughly. Precautionary measures were discussed and each subject was reminded that he/she could withdraw from the study at any time.

Subjects in all groups were also assigned to one of ten teams that worked closely with one another throughout the program. A phone chain was established within each team to develop a strong link with the coordinator. Each subject was assigned another person to phone daily to voice concerns or questions that might have developed. The phone chain culminated with a team leader who phoned the coordinator each evening. Team meetings were scheduled weekly for the first six weeks and then every other week until termination of the study. Weekly distances walked by each subject were recorded at team meetings. At the final meeting, all subjects in all groups were asked to fill out the questionnaire again re-assessing self perception of life satisfaction and health status. Further, each subject scheduled an appointment with his/her physician during the week following the completion of the study. Again, each physician was asked to rate the patient's health status.

RESULTS

Two 2 x 3 ANOVAs were computed blocking on sex and experimental condition with life satisfaction scores serving as the dependent variables for one and health status serving as the dependent variable for the other. As shown in Table 1, a significant F ratio was calculated for the condition main effect. As depicted in Table 3, a Scheffe post hoc analysis demonstrated significantly higher life satisfaction mean values for the walking-alone and walking-in-pairs groups (M=2.96, M=3.15, respectively) versus the control group (M=1.90). Although the walking-in-pairs group demonstrated a larger mean value than the walking-alone group, no significant difference was found. Further, no significant difference was elicited for the sex main effect or the interaction.

The results of the second ANOVA, as shown in Table 2, also demonstrated a significant main effect for condition. As depicted in Table 4, the results of the Scheffe post hoc test demonstrated that the walking conditions again elicited significantly higher health status mean values (M=2.70, M=2.90, respectively) versus the control condition (M=1.78). No significant difference was demonstrated for the sex main effect or the interaction.

DISCUSSION

The improvement in self-assessed life satisfaction and health status for the walking condition groups provides support for a positive effect of physical exercise. Some researchers have reported non-significant changes in life satisfaction among their subjects after an exercise regimen (Ray et al., 1983; Sidney & Shephard, 1976; Gutman et al., 1977). The results of this study may be attributed to the subject selection process prior to exercise initiation. The positive psychosocial and health status changes found in this study lend support to other investigations in which improved self esteem and alteration of mood and personality were found (Hanson & Nedde, 1974; Massie & Sheppard, 1971). Further, the discovery that those subjects who walked in pairs rated both life satisfaction and health status higher than those who walked alone should be emphasized. It is obvious that exercising in pairs had a distinct impact on the self assessments; however, further investigation is necessary.

In addition to the self-assessed changes documented, it is important to note the very interesting observations made by personal physicians at the termination of the exercise program. Eighty-two percent of the subjects' physicians reported an increase in patient health status. Other remarks by physicians included: patient weight loss, reduction in blood pressure, and an observable increase in morale.

Further investigation is necessary to examine adherence to exercise regimens by individuals who have made positive changes in health status and life satisfaction. Also, continued investigation is necessary into the social parameters displayed by subjects walking in pairs.

REFERENCES

Benestad, A.M. (1965). Trainability of old men. *Acta Med. Scand., 178,* 321-327.

Blue, F.R. (1979). Aerobic running as a treatment for moderate depression. *Perceptual and Motor Skills, 49,* 2.

de Vries, H.A. (1970). Physiological effects of an exercise training regiment upon men aged 52-88. *Journal of Gerontology, 25,* 325-336.

Edwards, J. & Klemmack, D. (1973). Correlates of life satisfaction: A re-examination. *Journal of Gerontology, 28,* 484-492.

Gutman, G., Herbert, C. & Brown, S. (1977). Feldenkrais versus conventional exercises for the elderly. *Journal of Gerontology, 32,* 562-572.

Hammett, V. (1967). Psychological changes with physical fitness training. *Canadian Medical Association Journal, 96,* 764-767.

Hansen, G. & Yoshioka, R. (1962). *Aging in the upper midwest: A profile of 6,300 senior citizens.* Community Studies, Kansas City.

Hanson, J. & Nedde, W. (1974). Long-term physical training effect in sedentary females. *Journal of Applied Physiology, 32,* 562-572.

Harris, R. & Frankel, L. (1977). *Guide to Fitness After Fifty.* New York: Plenum Press.

Kavanaugh, T., Shephard, R., Koney, H., & Pandit, V. (1973). Exercise in coronary rehabilitation. *Medicine and Science in Sports, 5,* 34-39.

Kennedy, C., King, J. & Muraco, W. (1983). The relative strength of health as a predictor of life satisfaction. *International Social Science, 58,* 97-102.

King, J. & Muraco, W. (1980). Needs assessment study of the aging adult. Northwest Ohio Council on Aging: Community Study.

Mancini, J. (1980). Effects of health and income on control orientation and life satisfaction among aged public housing residents. *International Journal of Aging and Human Development, 12,* 215-219.

Markides, K. & Martin, H. (1979). A causal model of life satisfaction among the elderly. *Journal of Gerontology, 34,* 86-93.

Massie, J. & Shephard, R. (1971). Physiological and psychological effects of training. *Medicine and Science in Sports, 3,* 110-117.

Neugarten, B., Havighurst, R. & Tobin, S. (1961). The measure of life satisfaction. *Journal of Gerontology, 16,* 134-143.

Palmore, E. & Kivett, V. (1977). Change in life satisfaction: A longitudinal study of persons aged 45-70. *Journal of Gerontology, 32,* 311-316.

Powell, R. (1974). Psychological effects of exercise therapy upon institutionalized geriatric mental patients. *Journal of Gerontology, 29,* 157-161.

Ray, R., Gissal, M. & Smith, E. (1983). The effect of exercise on morale of older adults. *Physical and Occupational Therapy in Geriatrics, 2,* 53-62.

Sidney, K. & Shephard, R. (1977b). Activity patterns of elderly men and women. *Journal of Gerontology, 32,* 25-32.

Sonquist, J., Baker, E. & Morgan, J. (1973). *Searching for structure.* Institute for Social Research, University of Michigan, Ann Arbor, Michigan.

Spreitzer, E. & Larson, D. (1979). Predictors of life satisfaction. *International Journal of Aging and Human Development, 10,* 283-288.

Spreitzer, E. & Snyder, E. (1974). Correlates of life satisfaction among the aged. *Journal of Gerontology, 29,* 454-458.

Stamford, B., Hambacher, W. & Fallica, A. (1974). Effects of daily physical exercise on the psychiatric state of institutionalized geriatric mental patients. *Research Quarterly, 45,* 34-41.

Table 1. Two-way analysis of variance for life satisfaction.

Source	df	SS	MS	F	p
Condition	2	44.31	22.16	80.28	.00*
Sex	1	.06	.06	.00	.96
CS	2	.02	.01	.05	.89
Error	139	38.36	.28		

*p < .05

Table 2. Two-way analysis of variance for health status.

Source	df	SS	MS	F	p
Condition	2	33.03	16.52	57.71	.00*
Sex	1	.25	.24	.87	.35
CS	2	.36	.18	.63	.54
Error	139	39.78	.29		

*p < .05

Table 3. Scheffe Post Hoc Analysis for life satisfaction treatment effect.

Condition	Control (M = 1.90)	Alone (M = 2.96)	Pairs (M = 3.15)
Control		1.06*	1.25*
Alone			.19

*p < .05

Note. SSR = .26

Table 4. Scheffe Post Hoc Analysis for health status treatment effect.

Condition	Control ($\underline{M} = 1.78$)	Alone ($\underline{M} = 2.70$)	Pairs ($\underline{M} = 2.90$)
Control		.92*	1.12*
Alone			.20

*$\underline{p} < .05$

Note. SSR = .27

10

EFFECTS OF AGE, GENDER, AND PERSONALITY ON PREVENTIVE HEALTH BEHAVIORS

Rickard A. Sebby
William E. Snell, Jr.

The relationship between preventive health behaviors and health-related aspects of personality were examined among 289 individuals aged 18 to 83, using separate measures of preventive health behaviors and personality tendencies. Hierarchical multiple regression analyses indicated that both health-anxiety and health-esteem affected health promoting behaviors, with these relationships moderated by age and gender. The discussion focuses on the need for educational programs tailored to the specific needs of particular age groups of males and females.

As the average age of our population increases, preventive health behaviors have been increasingly studied owing to the increasing costs associated with the health care of older individuals. Research has principally focused upon young and middle-aged adults (e.g., Harris & Guten, 1979), although evidence describing health practices among the elderly is accumulating (e.g., Amir, 1987; Bausell, 1986; Palmore, 1970). The findings from these studies suggest that elderly individuals may be more health conscious than the rest of the population (e.g., Bausell, 1986) and that the elderly engage in a wide range of behaviors that could be defined as preventive or health seeking (Amir, 1987). However, the causes for such increased consciousness and preventive behavior have not been adequately explored.

Various demographic factors (e.g., age, gender) have been examined in relation to the tendency to engage in health preventive behavior. Harris and Guten (1979) found that age was only weakly correlated with selected preventive behaviors. A review by Norman (1985) indicates that women have been found to engage in more preventive behaviors than men, although this relationship is not consistently indicated.

Personality is another aspect which has also been linked to physical well-being and health. Wallston and Wallston (1978, 1982) and Wallston, Smith, King, Forsberg, Wallston, and Nagy (1983) have found that health locus of control is associated with one's orientation toward health. Other personality characteristics (e.g., health esteem and confidence, motivation to avoid unhealthiness) have also been found to be related to preventive health behaviors in a recent study by Snell, Johnson, Lloyd, and Hoover (in press). However, these studies did not examine the relationship between personality factors, preventive health behaviors, age, or gender.

The present investigation examined the nature of the relationship between preventive health behaviors and personality factors related to health among males and females aged 18 to 83. Although previous research has indicated that health promoting or preventive health behavior tends to increase across the life span (Bausell, 1986) and that personality variables do affect the tendency to engage in preventive behavior (Snell et al., in press), a life-span examination of this relationship has not been previously conducted. It was anticipated that males and females at varying age levels would differ with respect to those personality variables which would be related to preventive health behaviors.

METHOD

Subjects

Two hundred and eighty-nine subjects (86 males and 203 females) between the ages of 18 and 83 participated in this study. All of the subjects were living independently in a middle-sized midwestern USA community.

Instruments

Two instruments were administered to all subjects. The Health Orientation Scale (HOS) consists of 10 health-related personality tendencies previously validated in a study by Snell et al. (in press): *private health consciousness,* defined as the tendency to be highly aware of and to think about one's physical health-fitness; *health image concern,* defined as the tendency to be highly aware of the external, observable impression that one's physical health makes on others; *health anxiety,* defined as the tendency to be anxious and nervous about one's physical health-fitness; *health esteem,* defined as a generalized tendency to positively evaluate and to feel confident about one's physical health; *motivation to avoid unhealthiness,* defined as the motivation and desire to avoid being in a state of unhealthiness; *motivation for healthiness,* defined as the motivational tendency and desire to keep oneself in good physical health; *internal health control,* defined as the tendency to believe that one's physical health and fitness is a direct function of one's own behaviors and actions; *external health control,* defined as the tendency to believe that one's health status is determined by uncontrollable factors external to oneself; *health expectations,* defined as the tendency to optimistically expect that one's health will be excellent and positive in the future; and *health status,* defined as the tendency to regard oneself as being currently well-exercised and in good physical shape. Subjects responded to the 50 items measuring these health-related personality factors on a 5-point Likert scale, higher scores corresponding to more of each tendency.

The second instrument, a measure of preventive health behaviors, was developed by Bausell (1986) and consisted of seven dietary factors, four safety practices, two health monitoring acts, and six general life-style variables. Responses on the measure of health-promoting behaviors were summed across the items with higher scores indicating a greater number of health seeking behaviors. (Due to an error in the construction of the item dealing with alcohol consumption, data from only 19 items were included in the resulting sum.) The items were scored "1" if the respondents indicated engaging in the behaviors (otherwise a "0").

RESULTS

Subjects' scores on the HOS were compiled for each of the 10 subscales. The means for these subscales as well as for the healthy behavior index are presented in Table 1. An inspection of this table indicates that as a group the subjects were characterized by a positive outlook toward their health. For example, they were quite conscious of health concerns, had an internal health locus of control, and were optimistic about the future status of their health. In addition, it can be seen in Table 1 that the subjects reported that they engaged in a considerable number of preventive health behaviors (an average of 12.56 out of 19).

Hierarchical multiple regression analyses were performed to determine whether health promoting behavior was predicted by age (linear and quadratic effects), the 10 subscale scores of the HOS, and the interaction effects associated with these variables. Separate analyses were conducted for each gender. In the first step of each set of analyses, the main effects of age (linear and quadratic) and the ten HOS subscales were entered. The second step consisted of entering the interaction effects according to the predictive value each effect contributed to the regression equation.

Examination of the resulting regression equation for males indicated an R of .61 (p<.001), with the following variables having the greatest value for predicting health promoting behavior: motivation for healthiness (B=.57, p<.03), motivation to avoid unhealthiness (B=.39, p<.01), the age by health anxiety quadratic interaction effect (B=-1.27, p<.01), and the age by health-esteem quadratic interaction effect (B=-.65, p<.04).

The results obtained for females indicated that the regression equation had an R of .27 (p<.01) with the linear effect of age (B=.15, p<.05), the motivation to avoid unhealthiness (B=.25, p<.04), and the age by health-esteem quadratic interaction effect (B=-.17, p<.05) having significant predictive value.

These data do indicate some similarity between the responses of males and females. Both males and females were found to engage in more health seeking behaviors the greater their motivation to avoid unhealthiness. However, anxiety about one's health was found to significantly affect males' and not females' health promoting behaviors. Figure 1 indicates the nature of this finding. For males who were low in health anxiety, young and old males engaged in more health promoting behaviors relative to middle-aged males. Males high in health anxiety generally engaged in less health-promoting behaviors, with a linear decrease noted across increasing age levels.

The findings for the health-esteem by age interaction indicated two somewhat different patterns for males and females. These patterns are shown in Figure 2. *Males* who were high in health-esteem generally engaged in more health promoting behaviors than did those who had lower health-esteem levels, with levels of health promoting behavior gradually declining across age. Middle-aged males, as compared with those classified as young and old, engaged in fewer health promoting behaviors.

For *females* the nature of the age-by-health esteem interaction assumed a different nature. Among those reporting a high level of health-esteem, middle-aged females had the highest levels of health promoting behavior, with older women falling below young women. A general linear increase in health promoting behavior was noted for women having lower levels of health-esteem.

DISCUSSION

The results of this study provide evidence that health-related personality tendencies influence the extent to which people engaged in health promoting behaviors across the life span. The research evidence indicated that higher levels of health-anxiety depress health promoting behavior among males. By contrast, lower levels of health-anxiety generally lead to more preventive health behavior, although for middle-aged males who are in the midst of career pursuits, this low level of health-anxiety may lessen their perceived need for engaging in such health sustaining behaviors. Health-esteem was also found to influence people's tendency to engage in health promoting behaviors, although the nature of the relationship differed for males and females. The findings that older women with higher levels of health-esteem engage in fewer health seeking behaviors may indicate that the perceived need for such behaviors is not recognized by these women (perhaps due to chronological or cohort-related attitudes). For males, higher health-esteem is positively related to the tendency to engage in healthy behaviors across the life span. Low esteem by contrast seems to depress pursuits of health-related behavior, particularly among middle-aged males.

In conclusion, the present findings revealed that health-related personality tendencies influence men's and women's tendency to engage in health promoting behaviors, with the relationship being moderated by their chronological age. As such, it is apparent that these data indicate that educational programs designed to help improve people's health need to be tailored to specific age ranges for males and females. Specifically, educational programs addressing cohort-related attitudes which act to diminish preventative health behaviors among groups of older females may need to be designed even though these individuals may outwardly express few concerns about their health. For males the focus of such educational efforts may need to be on raising their health-esteem in order to facilitate the acquisition of preventative health behaviors. Middle age men with low health-anxiety would seem to be another significant target group which may be particularly in need of specific educational programs designed to raise their general health values, sensitize them to the possibility and preventability of diseases likely to affect their particular group, an to inform them of the consequences of such disorders if not prevented (Taylor, 1986).

The psychology of personality and individual tendencies is an important aspect of understanding health-related behavior, and the study of these psychological tendencies is vital to the promotion of preventive health behaviors and compliance with recommended health practices. As a result, it is important that much more emphasis be placed on an examination of these tendencies as they may manifest themselves among males and females in various age groups. At this time the Health Orientation

Scale (HOS; Snell et al., in press) is one of the few available omnibus instruments that comprehensively assesses a wide variety of personality and individual tendencies associated with health and fitness. We would argue that this objective self-report instrument merits further research use. It can provide personality researchers and health practitioners with a comprehensive approach to the study of health, and if used appropriately it can increase our understanding of health-related behaviors.

Portions of this article were presented at the 1989 annual meeting of the American Psychological Association, New Orleans, Louisiana, U.S.A.

REFERENCES

Amir, D. (1987). Preventive behavior and health status among the elderly. *Psychology and Health: An International Journal, 1*, 353-378.

Bausell, R.B. (1986). Health-seeking behavior among the elderly. *The Gerontologist, 26*, 556-559.

Harris, D. & Guten, S. (1979). Health protective behavior: An exploratory study. *Journal of Health and Social Behavior, 20*, 17-29.

Norman, R. (1985). *The nature and correlates of health behavior.* Health Promotion Studies No. 2. Ottawa: Health Promotion Directorate.

Palmore, E. (1970). Health practices and illness among the aged. *The Gerontologist, 10*, 313-316.

Snell, W.E., Jr., Johnson, G., Lloyd, P.J. & Hoover, M.W. (in press). The development and validation of the Health Orientation Scale: A measure of psychological tendencies associated with health. *European Journal of Personality.*

Taylor, S.E. (1986). *Health Psychology.* New York: Random House.

Wallston, K.A., Smith, R.A., King, J.E., Forsberg, P.R., Wallston, B.S. & Nagy, V.T. (1983). Expectancies about control over health: Relationship to desire for control of health care. *Personality and Social Psychology Bulletin, 9,* 377-385.

Wallston, K.A. & Wallston, B.S. (1978). Locus of control and health: A review of the literature. *Health Education Monographs, 6,* 107-117.

Wallston, K.A. & Wallston, B.S. (1982). Who is responsible for your health? The construct of health locus of control. In G. Sanders and J. Suls (Eds.) *Social psychology of health and illness.* Hillsdale, NJ: Lawrence Erlbaum and Associates.

Table 1

Means and Standard Deviations on the HOS and Bausell's (1986) Preventive Health Behaviors Instrument

Measures	Mean	SD
1. Personal Health Consciousness	14.59	3.94
2. Health Image Concern	8.83	5.60
3. Health Anxiety	8.08	4.56
4. Health Esteem-Confidence	12.12	4.23
5. Motivation to Avoid Unhealthiness	12.72	4.22
6. Motivation for Healthiness	12.15	4.46
7. Internal Health Control	15.36	.3.95
8. External Health Control	5.47	3.98
9. Health Expectations	12.76	4.18
10. Health Status	10.92	4.34
11. Health Promoting Behaviors	12.56	3.22

Note. Higher scores on the HOS subscales indicate a greater degree of each of the health-related tendencies (range = 0-20). Higher scores on Bausell's measure indicates a greater tendency to report engaging in health promoting behaviors (range = 0-19).

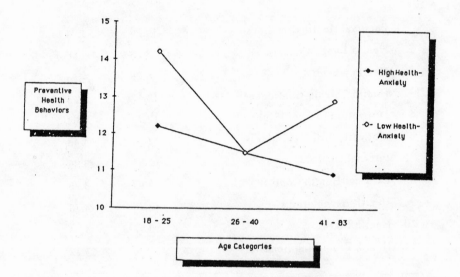

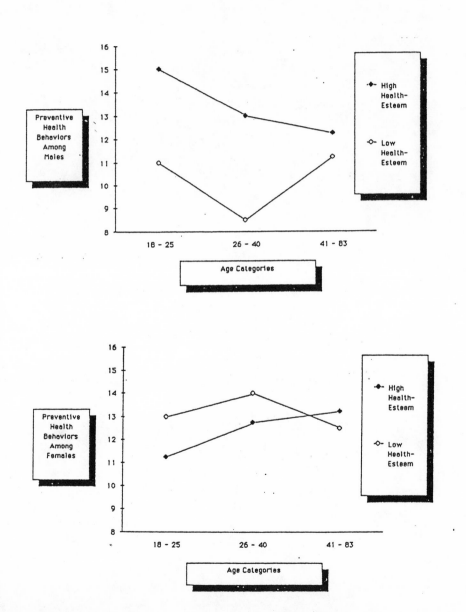

11

ARGENTINE HEMORRHAGIC FEVER: THE RELATIONSHIP OF SOCIAL SUPPORT AND OTHER PSYCHOSOCIAL FACTORS TO PREVENTIVE HEALTH BEHAVIORS

Josefa Ippolito-Shepherd
Robert H. L. Feldman
Roberta B. Hollander

Argentine Hemorrhagic Fever (AHF) is a viral disease which infects rural workers in the most populous region of Argentina. With a fatality rate of 5 to 30%, it is a major public health problem. To understand the relationship of social support and other psychosocial factors to preventing and controlling AHF, the present study was conducted. A sample of 306 participants in 12 towns completed questionnaires which examined their intention to wear protective clothing, control weeds in residential and work areas, and seek early treatment when experiencing AHF symptoms. The results indicate that social support was utilized most for weed control (a communal responsibility) and early treatment, and less for protective clothing (a personal responsibility). Also, other psychosocial factors, including attitudes, subjective norm, knowledge and information, contributed to our understanding of AHF preventive health behaviors.

The concept of social support associated with health and well-being has attracted increasing attention. This is apparent in the growing body of literature on social support and in its use in health promotion and education interventions (Cohen & Syme, 1985; Sarason, Sarason & Pierce, 1990; Schwarzer & Leppin, 1989).

Social support has been conceptualized as valued feedback provided by primary group members and peers (Gottlieb, 1985; Cassel, 1976). Social support persons may facilitate the ability of the individual to mobilize psychological resources and gain control over an emotional burden (Caplan, 1974). Persons who are part of an individual's social support group or network share tasks with that individual, and may provide money, materials, skills and counseling to enhance the person's capacity to handle a situation (Caplan, 1974).

A variety of settings conducive to the delivery of social support have been studied, including worksites, physicians' offices, homes (visits by health workers), and dental offices. There is consistent evidence across many physical disorders, that naturally recurring support is beneficial, while social isolation is not (Haynes, Taylor & Sackett, 1979; Wallston, et al., 1983).

Among the research that has documented the beneficial effects of social support is a study measuring the impact of stressors and social support on the outcome of pregnancy (Nuckolls et al., 1972). This study found that women with low social support were more likely to experience complications than women with high social support.

Social support in the form of social networks has also been noted to influence the use of health services. In a twelve-month prospective longitudinal study on the use of pediatric acute care services by 513 children and their families enrolled in a prepaid group practice, in addition to the child's age, birth order, baseline health status, and ethnic group, social networks were found to be important predictors of acute care utilization. The study showed significant effects for network size, dispersion and the tendency to use one's network members. Individuals with large nondispersed networks were most likely to use pediatric health services. The tendency to call on network members was noted to modify an individual's propensity to seek care for minor pediatric medical problems (Horwitz, Morgenstern & Berkman, 1985).

A nine-year mortality follow-up study of 17,000 adults in Alameda County, California indicated that morbidity and mortality rates from all causes were related to a composite index of social ties. Persons who had few ties to other people exhibited mortality rates two to five times higher than those with more ties, even when traditional risk factors were controlled (Berkman & Syme, 1979).

Research about the effects of social support has been plagued with a variety of problems. First, the conceptualization of social support varies, which undermines its specific meaning and limits its validity. Five dimensions of social support (intimacy, social integration, nurturance, alliance, and guidance) (Weiss, 1974), and three types of social support (personal, intraorganizational, and extraorganizational) (Kelly, Munoz & Snowden, 1979) have been identified. However, it has been suggested that despite variations in how social support is conceptualized, it would seem to have two basic elements: a perceived number of, and a degree of satisfaction with available support persons (Sarason et al., 1983).

Second, a barrier to research has been the lack of a reliable and convenient measure (Sarason et al., 1983). Studies in this area have focused largely on specific aspects of social support without necessarily identifying key elements essential to a reliable index. For example, some studies (Miller & Ingram, 1976; Miller, Ingram & Davidson, 1976), have identified only who the individual's confidants and acquaintances were or the availability of "helpful others" in coping with certain work, family, and financial problems (Medalie & Goldbourt, 1976). Some effort has been made to include these key elements in instruments. For example, a 50-question structured interview has been developed to measure the perceived availability and adequacy of people who can be counted on for assistance in problem-solving and emotional support, and to measure the availability and adequacy of social integration (Henderson, 1980); and a measure has been designed to assess the frequency with which people are the recipients of supportive actions (Barrera, Sandler & Ramsay, 1981). Studies have also been conducted that provide information about the relationships and correlates of dimensions of social support with other measures, such as desirable and undesirable life events, perceived adequacy of childhood relationships, personality characteristics, and outlook about the future (Sarason et al., 1983).

The concept of social support, then, implies a pattern of ties that plays a significant part in maintaining the psychological and physical integrity of the individual. Social support may be regarded as a cushion against the harmful effects of stressful life changes, with the support as a modifier in the stressor-illness relationship (Cassel, 1974; Cassel, 1976; Cobb, 1976; Kaplan, Cassel & Gore, 1977; Lin, Woelfel & Light, 1985; Nuckolls et al., 1972). It is also likely that the absence of support is a stressor in itself, and as such has a direct influence on a person's health status (Thoits, 1982).

Although significant advances have been made to provide greater understanding of the role of social support in health issues, additional research is warranted. The present study is an effort of this order.

ARGENTINE HEMORRHAGIC FEVER (AHF)

The Federal Republic of Argentina, located in southeastern South America, is the second largest Latin American country and has an estimated population of 31 million people (U.S. Department of State, 1990). Argentina is primarily an agricultural country, with most of its products from the AHF endemic area encompassing the provinces of Buenos Aires, La Pampa, Santa Fe and Cordoba. This area is the most populous in the country (Mettler, 1969).

AHF was first recognized in the 1950s in the northwest Buenos Aires province of Argentina (Mettler, 1969). The etiologic agent, the Junin virus, a member of the Arenaviridiae, was isolated and named in 1958 (Pasqualini, 1977). The virus has been found to infect persistently several species of field mice. Among these, the Calomys musculinus is suspected to be the main reservoir (Acha & Szyfres, 1986; Weissenbacher & Damonte, 1983).

AHF affects mostly male rural workers engaged in harvesting crops. The disease appears to be transmitted through the rodent's saliva and urine. The virus is thought to reach the person mucosally or cutaneously (Acha & Szyfres, 1986). Transmission between humans is exceptional, but the virus has been reported to have been isolated from pharyngeal swabs and from the urine of sick patients (Acha & Szyfres, 1986; Benenson, 1990; Weissenbacher & Damonte, 1983).

Infected persons exhibit cardiovascular, renal, hematological, and digestive involvement, as well as central nervous system disorders, in varying degrees of severity. A fatality rate of 5 to 30% has been found. The reported number of cases peaks in mid-autumn (April to June), at the same time that the rodent population increases. Early immunoserum treatment has been shown to reduce the mortality rates (Benenson, 1990; Maiztegui, Fernandez & Damilano, 1982; Weissenbacher & Damonte, 1983).

The prevention and control of AHF requires reducing the size of the rodent population, minimizing human contact with the rodents, and early detection and treatment of infected persons. Because of the characteristics of the endemic region, it is very difficult to reduce the rodent population. Immunization would result in protecting the susceptible population, but at the time of this study, a live attenuated vaccine was under development. Treatment with immunoserum (immunoglobulin) within eight days of the first symptoms can markedly reduce the mortality rate (Maiztegui, Fernandez & Damilano, 1979).

Accordingly, at this time the risks associated with AHF can be decreased through health education programs that increase knowledge of the etiology of the disease and promote attitudes and personal behaviors conducive to preventing and controlling AHF. Health education programs have been implemented in the area, but their effectiveness had not been evaluated at the time this study was undertaken (Ippolito-Shepherd, 1984). These programs were mostly ad hoc lectures until 1984 when a mass media program was launched in several regions of the endemic area (Ippolito-Shepherd et al., 1987). The program promoted the use of protective clothing, weed control, and early diagnosis and treatment of AHF.

The study presented here examined the perceived availability of social support to carry out these behaviors, and the intention of study participants to adopt the behaviors as predicted by their perceptions of their social support systems. Additionally, this study explored the predictive value of attitudes, subjective norms, knowledge, and information to adopt behaviors to prevent and control AHF.

METHOD

The population that participated in this study consisted of 306 rural inhabitants over 18 years of age who lived in the endemic area of AHF and who volunteered to take part in the survey. Twelve towns were selected for inclusion in the study based on AHF epidemiological characteristics. The selected towns had a minimum of 50 km distance between them. The population was asked to participate in this survey by representatives of the local agricultural cooperatives, who either visited the individual households or informed people when they visited the agricultural cooperatives. The sample selected was a convenience sample. The minimum requirements for inclusion in the sample were that participants be over 18 years of age and that they were residents of the 12 towns selected. Volunteers for the study were requested to meet at assigned locations at specified times to complete the survey instrument.

The format for the questionnaire was adopted from the Theory of Reasoned Action Model (Ajzen & Fishbein, 1980). The self-administered questionnaire in Spanish consisted of a total of 74 items, of which 12 were for behavioral intention, 12 for attitude toward behavior, 12 for subjective norms, 12 for social support, 14 for knowledge, three for information sources, and the remaining questions elicited sociodemographic data. A three-point scale format was used for all items except for the questions on the information component, which utilized a multiple choice format, and the sociodemographic items, which were to be filled in by respondents. The instrument was pretested in the AHF area with 34 rural inhabitants with characteristics similar to the target population, and was revised accordingly.

For purposes of this study, protective clothing is a composite term that included gloves, boots, long pants/skirts, and long-sleeved shirts which were recommended as personal preventive measures to diminish the risk of the virus infecting persons through skin cuts or abrasions on the hands, arms, or legs.

Weed control is a composite term that included cutting back high weeds in the residential and work areas. This measure is recommended to eliminate or at least decrease the hiding places of rodents that are the reservoir of the Junin virus.

Early treatment is a composite term that included seeking early diagnosis and treatment if experiencing symptoms common to AHF (i.e., fever, weakness, headaches, leg or abdominal pain, or dizziness-nausea). Early diagnosis and treatment are recommended to reduce the risk of further morbidity and of dying as a result of this disease.

RESULTS

Of the 306 persons, 52 participants were females and 254 were males. Ninety-six percent of the sample had been born in Argentina, and 90% had lived in the same town for more than 12 years. Ninety-two percent owned their own homes, and all except one person had some formal education.

Ninety percent of the study participants reported that they had received information with respect to AHF. Seventy-four percent received their information from television, 70% from radio, and 51% from newspapers/magazines. Eighty-three percent of the participants responded with a 70% accuracy to the items pertaining to the etiology and methods of prevention and control of AHF.

Perceived social support for all protective clothing items was reported by 19.6% of the people surveyed. The percentage for each item was 21.9% for boots, 21.9% for long pants/skirts, 23.2% for long sleeved shirts, and 24.2% for gloves (Table 1). All weed control items was reported by 29.7% (31.4% for around the work area and 35.6% for around the living area). For all early treatment items, perceived social support was reported by 28.1% of participants, including 32.4% for headaches, 35.0% for weakness, 36.3% for leg pain, 39.5% for fever, and 40.8% for dizziness-nausea.

As Table 2 indicates, multiple regression analysis revealed the following:

Protective Clothing

The F value for behavior intention for protective clothing was significant in relation to the predictor variables tested (F=10.29, p<0.001). The standardized estimates were significant for attitude (b=0.14, p<0.01), subjective norm (b=0.21, p<0.001), social support (b=0.21, p<0.001), and knowledge (b=0.14, p<0.01). The standardized estimate for information was nonsignificant at p=0.05. The squared multiple correlation for this equation was R^2=0.15, and the stepwise regression entered these predictor variables into the equation in the following order: subjective norm (R^2=0.07), social support (R^2=0.04), attitude (R^2=0.02), and knowledge (R^2=0.02).

Weed Control

The F value for behavior intention for weed control was significant in relation to the predictor variables tested (F=13.07, p<0.001). The standardized estimates were significant for only two of the five predictor variables tested: attitudes (b=0.34, p<0.001) and knowledge (b=0.11, p<0.05). The squared multiple correlation coefficient for this equation was R^2=0.18, and the stepwise regression entered the independent variables into the equation as attitude (R^2=0.15), subjective norm (R^2=0.01), and knowledge (R^2=0.01).

Early Treatment

The F value for behavior intention for early treatment was significant in relation to the five predictor variables tested (F=30.46, p<0.001). All predictor variables showed significant standardized estimates except for knowledge. These were: attitude (b=0.40, p<0.001), subjective norm (b=0.14, p<0.01), social support (b=0.20, p<0.001), and information (b=0.16, p<0.001). The squared multiple correlation coefficient for this equation was R^2=0.34, and the stepwise regression entered the predictor variables studied as attitude (R^2=0.24), social support (R^2=0.04), information (R^2=0.03), and subjective norm (R^2=0.02).

DISCUSSION

The purposes of this paper were twofold: first, to assess and describe the perceived availability of social support associated with behaviors conducive to the prevention and control of AHF, and second, to assess and describe the predictive value of perceived social support, attitudes, subjective norms, knowledge and information on the intention to carry out the specified behaviors.

The data showed that the study participants were similar with respect to their place of birth, living conditions, educational level and exposure to, and knowledge about AHF and its methods of prevention and control. The perceived availability of social support was found to be highest for weed control (29.7%) and early treatment (28.1%), and lowest for protective clothing (19.6%). The perceived social support for early diagnosis and treatment also varied proportionately with the severity of the symptoms. For example, dizziness-nausea exhibited the highest perceived social support (40.8%) compared with headaches as the lowest (32.4%). The low level of perceived social support for the use of protective clothing may be due to the personal nature of this behavior and the fact that the behavior takes place prior to the appearance of symptoms when the individual assessment of personal susceptibility to AHF, severity of the disease, and perceived benefits of the preventive behaviors may be weakest. This is in contrast to weed control, which, in addition to being a control measure, may involve a sense of communal responsibility, and early diagnosis and treatment which takes place once symptoms are evident.

Thus, in regard to the first purpose of this study, participants showed perceived social support for the behaviors conducive to the prevention and control of AHF. Future activities that address preventive measures for AHF need to take into account the specific elements of social support of the target population in order to achieve the objective for these activities.

With respect to the second purpose, the multiple regression analysis showed that perceived social support was a significant predictor for the intention to wear protective clothing and for early diagnosis, but not for weed control. Attitude was a significant predictor for behavior intention to wear protective clothing, for

224 *Ippolito-Shepherd, Feldman and Hollander*

weed control, and for early diagnosis and treatment. The highest predictive value of attitude for early diagnosis and treatment may be attributed to the perceived susceptibility to AHF after the symptoms are evident.

Other psychosocial factors which significantly predicted behavioral intent were subjective norm, knowledge, and information. Therefore, this set of psychosocial factors contributed to our understanding of AHF preventive health behaviors.

REFERENCES

Acha, P.N. & Szyfres, B. (1986). Zoonoses and communicable diseases common to man and animals (Scientific Publication No. 503). Washington, D.C.: Pan American Health Organization, World Health Organization.

Ajzen, I. & Fishbein, M. (1980). *Understanding attitudes and predicting social behavior.* Englewood Cliffs, New Jersey: Prentice-Hall.

Berrera, M., Jr., Sandler, I.N. & Ramsay, T.B. (1981). Preliminary development of a scale of social support: Studies on college students. *American Journal of Community Psychology, 9,* 435-447.

Benenson, A.S. (Ed.) (1985). *Social support and health.* Orlando, Florida: Academic Press, Inc.

Benenson, A.S. (Ed.) (1990). *Control of communicable diseases in man.* (15th ed.) Washington, D.C.: The American Public Health Association.

Berkman, L.F. & Syme, S.L. (1979). Social networks, host resistance, and mortality: A nine-year follow-up study of Alameda County residents. *American Journal of Epidemiology, 109,* (2), 186-204.

Caplan, G. (1974). *Support systems and community mental health.* New York: Human Sciences Press.

Cassel, J. (1976). The contribution of the social environment to host resistance. *American Journal of Epidemiology, 104,* 107.

Cassel, J. (1974). An epidemiological perspective of psychosocial factors in disease etiology. *American Journal of Public Health, 64,* 1040.

Cobb, S. (1976). Social support as a moderator of life stress. *Journal of Psychosomatic Medicine, 38,* 300-314.

Gottlieb, B.H. (1985). Social networks and social support: An overview of research practice, and policy implications. *Health Education Quarterly, 12,* (1), 5-22.

Haynes, R.B., Taylor, D.W., & Sackett, D.L. (Eds.) (1979). *Compliance in health care.* Baltimore: The Johns Hopkins University Press.

Henderson, S. (1980). A development in social psychiatry: The systematic study of social bonds. *Journal of Nervous and Mental Disease, 168,* 63-69.

Horwitz, S., Morgenstern, H., & Berkman, L.F. (1985). The impact of social stressors and social networks on pediatric medical care use. *Medical Care, 23,* (8), 946-959.

Ippolito-Shepherd, J. (1984). *Argentine Hemorrhagic Fever: An Updated Bibliography.* A report to the PAHO, Washington, D.C. Pan American Health Organization, World Health Organization.

Ippolito-Shepherd, J., Feldman, R.H.L., Acha, P.N., Maiztegui, Castro, C. & Feuillade de Sensi, M.R. (1987). Agricultural occupational health and health education in Latin America and the Caribbean. *Health Education Research, 2,* (11), 53-59.

Kaplan, B.H., Cassel, J.C., & Gore, S. (1977). Social support and health. *Medical Case, 15,* (5) (Supplement), 47-58.

Kelly, J.G., Munoz, R.E. & Snowden, L.R. (1979). Characteristics of community research projects and the implementation process. In Munoz, R.E., Snowden, L.R., and Kelly, J.G. (Eds.) *Social and psychological research in community settings.* San Francisco: Jossey Bass.

Lin, N., Woelfel, M.W., & Light, S.C. (1985). The buffering effect of social support subsequent to an important life event. *Journal of Health and Social Behavior, 26,* 247-263.

Maiztegui, J.I., Fernandez, N.J. & de Damilano, A.J. (1982). *Epidemiology and specific treatment of Argentine Hemorrhagic Fever.* In *Simposio internacional sobre arbovirus dos tropicos e febres hemorragicas* (pp. 245-250). Belem-Para-Brazil, 14a 18 de abril, 1980. Rio do Janero: Academia Brasileira de Cieneias.

Maiztegui, J.I., Fernandez, N.J., & de Damilano, A.J. (1979). Efficacy of immune plasma in treatment of Argentine Hemorrhagic Fever and association between treatment and a late neurological syndrome. *The Lancet, 8,* 1216-1217.

Medalie, J.H. & Goldbourt, D. (1976). Angina pectoris among 10,000 men: II psychosocial and other risk factors as evidenced by multivariate analysis of a five-year incidence study. *American Journal of Medicine, 60,* 910-921.

Mettler, N.E. (1969). *Argentine hemorrhagic fever: Current knowledge* (Scientific Publication No. 183). Washington, D.C.: Pan American Health Organization, World Health Organization.

Miller, P. & Ingham, J.G. (1976). Friends, confidants, and symptoms. *Social Psychiatry, 11,* 51-58.

Miller, P., Ingham, J.G., & Davidson, E. (1976). Life event symptoms and social support. *Journal of Psychosomatic Research, 20,* 515-522.

Nuckolls, K.B., Cassel, J.C. & Kaplan, B.H. (1972). Psychosocial assets, life crisis and the prognosis of pregnancy. *American Journal of Epidemiology, 95,* 341.

Pasqualini, C.D. (1977). Fiebres hemorragicas producida por Arenaviruses. *Medicina* (Buenos Aires) *37* (Suplemento 3), 1-2.

Sarason, I.G., Levine, H.M, Basham, R.B., & Sarason, B.R. (1983). Assessing social support: The social support questionnaire. *Journal of Personality and Social Psychology, 44,* (1), 127-139.

Sarason, B.R., Sarason, J.G., & Pierce, G.R. (1990). *Social support: An international view.* New York: John Wiley.

Schwarzer, R. & Leppin, A. (1989). Social support and health: A meta-analysis. *Psychology and Health, 3,* 1-15.

Thoits, P.A. (1982). Conceptual, methodological, and theoretical problems in studying social support as a buffer against life stress. *Journal of Health and Social Behavior, 23,* 145.

United States Department of State (1990). *Argentina: Background Notes* (Publication No. 7836). Washington, D.C.: Author.

Wallston, B.S., Alagha, S.W., DeVellis, B.M. & DeVellis, R.T. (1983). Social support and physical health. *Health Psychology, 2*, 41, 367-391.

Weiss, R.S. (1974). The provisions of social relations. In Rubin, Z. (Ed.) *Doing unto others.* Englewood Cliffs, New Jersey: Prentice-Hall.

Weissenbacher, M.C. & Damonte, E.B. (1983). Fiebre Hemorragica Argentina. *Adelantos Microbiologicos Enfermedades Infecciosas, 2*, 119-171.

Table 1: Perceived Social Support and

Preventive Health Behaviors (n=306)

Perceived Social Support (Percentage)

	No	I do not know	Yes
Protective Clothing	-	-	19.6*
Gloves	69.3	6.5	24.2
Boots	71.6	6.5	21.9
Long pants/skirt	72.2	.5.9	21.9
Long sleeves/shirt	71.9	4.9	23.2
Weed Control	-	-	29.7*
Living area	58.5	5.9	35.6
Work area	62.4	6.2	31.4
Early Treatment	-	-	28.1*
Fever	56.2	4.2	39.5
Weakness	60.8	4.2	35.0
Headaches	63.4	4.2	32.4
Leg pain	59.8	3.9	36.3
Dizziness-nausea	55.2	3.9	40.8

* Percentage of respondents who answered yes to all of the subitems of the behavior.

TABLE 2: Multiple Regression

Preventive Health Behavioral Intentions and Psychosocial Factors (n=306)

Criterion Variables	Predictor Variables	R Squared	Standardized Estimates
PROTECTIVE CLOTHING			
BEINTPC	ATBEHPC	0.02	0.14**
(Fvalue=10.29***)	SNBEHPC	0.07	0.21***
	SOSUPPC	0.04	0.21***
	KNOWLEDG	0.02	0.14**
	INFORMAT	0.00	-0.02
	Cumulative	0.15	
WEED CONTROL			
BEINTWC	ATBEHWC	0.15	0.34***
(Fvalue=13.07***)	SNBEHWC	0.01	0.09
	SOSUPWC	0.00	0.06
	KNOWLEDG	0.01	0.11*
	INFORMAT	0.00	0.02
	Cumulative	0.18	
EARLY TREATMENT			
BEINTET	ATBEHET	0.24	0.40***
(Fvalue=30.46***)	SNBEHET	0.02	0.14**
	SOSUPET	0.04	0.20***
	KNOWLED	0.00	0.04
	INFORMAT	0.03	0.16***
	Cumulative	0.34	

*   Significant p<0.05

**   Significant p<0.01

*** Significant p<0.001

BEINT   - Behavioral Intention

ATBEH   - Attitude

SNBEH   - Subjective Norm

SOSUP   - Social Support

KNOWLEDG - Knowledge

INFORMAT - Information

12

FACTORS PREDICTING INTENTION TO JOIN WORKSITE SMOKING-CESSATION PROGRAMS

M.C. Joelle Fignole Lofton
Robert H.L. Feldman

A social psychological model of health behavior was utilized to determine how well it predicted intent to join worksite smoking-cessation program. The model consisted of the psychosocial variables - social support, social norms, habit, self-efficacy, attitude, subjective norm, barriers, and behavioral intent. A total of 168 employees completed questionnaires measuring general intention to join and intention to join a specific program at the worksite. Forty respondents (23.8%) indicated they wanted to join the next available worksite program. Ethnicity and general intention explained 21% of the variance of specific intention, with Black employees expressing greater intention to join then White employees. Subjective norm, habit, and attitude explained 33.8% of the variance of general intention. A multivariate test of significance of six predictor variables (social norms and self-efficacy were excluded) and grade level at work differentiated between those intending and not intending to join a specific program (Hotellings $T^2=0.27$, $F[7,111]=4.23$, $p<.000$). A univariate test indicated the greater the general intention to join a program, the greater the specific intention to join ($F[1,117]=19.22$, $p<.000$). Results suggest the ethnic factor reflects a class and union membership difference and that worksite smoking-cessation programs sponsored by unions appeal more to lower income workers and union members.

The potential role of the workplace in promoting initiation and fostering the continuation of smoking behavior represents a kind of interaction between smoking and the workplace that may affect large numbers of U.S. workers. It seems clear that the responsibility for health in the workplace includes at minimum a work environment that does not promote smoking or interfere with cessation.
Everett Koop, M.D.

Over 30,000 studies link cigarette smoking to increased morbidity and mortality from cardiovascular diseases, various forms of cancer, and chronic obstructive lung disease (Klesges, Cigrang, and Glasgow, 1987). The authors cite studies indicating that cigarette smoking by employees results in increased expenses for both employers and employees. Klesges, Cigrang, and Glasgow also claim that smokers use the health care system up to 50% more than nonsmokers, which translates into higher health insurance costs for companies. Other studies have reported higher rates of work-related accidents, disability reimbursement payments, and absenteeism among employees who smoke compared to those who do not. Estimates of excess annual costs to employers per smoking employee generally run from $300 to $600. According to Klesges, Cigrang, and Glasgow (1987), these data as well as consideration for the welfare of employees, have led many businesses to establish workplace antismoking programs.

Klesges, Cigrang, and Glasgow (1987) claim approximately one-third of the adults in the United States smoke. Given this statistic, researchers of smoking cessation must begin to enlarge their framework in order to help smokers quit their habit. Specifically, researchers must look at the relationship of sociological and psychological factors and their interactive effect on an individual's ability to make health-related decisions and changes.

In this study we focused on the characteristics of smokers before they join programs. That is, by knowing which factors predict who joins smoking cessation programs, health educators can more adequately address the needs of joiners and accurately judge the likelihood for success.

We tested a set of variables based on the Feldman modification of the Wallston and Wallston (1984) unified social psychological model of health behavior. According to the Feldman model, behavior is a function of habit, intent (determined by attitudes and subjective norm), and self-efficacy (determined by barriers and social support). Tested by Quinn (1977), all of the variables contributed to the prediction of behavior. The variables in this model, plus an additional variable (social norms), were tested to ascertain their ability to predict who intends to join worksite smoking-cessation programs.

STUDIES ON JOINING SMOKING-CESSATION PROGRAMS

Brod and Hall (1984) compared psychosocial variables of joiners and nonjoiners in smoking treatment. The researchers found that joiners were less anxious, better educated, and had higher perceived self-efficacy than nonjoiners. Glasgow et al., (1987) studied predictors of participation and success in a worksite smoking-modification program and found older smokers who were heavier smokers were more likely to participate. However, Sussman et al., (1989) found the nonjoiners (of worksite smoking-cessation treatment) reported higher preprogram smoking levels.

Sussman et al., (1989) attempted to discriminate between joiners and nonjoiners of a smoking-cessation program based on the subject's own desire to quit or to not quit smoking. Among their findings: joiners reported significantly lower preprogram smoking levels, a lesser likelihood of having friends and children who smoked and greater self-efficacy to be able to stop smoking. Biener et al., (1987) cite an estimate that only 6% to 8% of smokers in moderate- to large-size companies participate in worksite smoking-cessation programs. In their study, the factors that differentiated the 28 joiners from the 85 nonjoiners included at least one prior quit attempt (93% versus 76%) and intention to quit in the next 6 months (78% versus 51%). Socioeconomic and demographic characteristics were found by Rost et al., (1987) to be the strongest predictors of participation in worksite health promotion programs. These characteristics explained 19% of the variance. Specifically, female and nonmanagement employees were more likely to participate.

Behavioral Intent

Behavioral intent, a person's belief that he or she will perform a particular behavior, is best described by Ajzen and Fishbein (1980). Fishbein (1982) stated that most behaviors of social relevance are under volitional control. Therefore a person's intention to perform (or not perform) a specific behavior is a major determinant of that action. Fishbein further assumes that barring unforeseen events, a person's intention should permit highly accurate predictions of his or her behavior. Sussman et al., (1989) state that a person's behavioral expectation of quitting would be a good predictor of whether he or she would join a smoking cessation clinic in the first place. Research shows that an item assessing the likelihood that a smoker would quit smoking at a specific time is an excellent predictor of quitting and relapse. In another study, the more successful abstainers believed that they would not be smoking in five years (Eisinger, 1971). In this study of predictors of smoking recidivism, this intention was one of the three most parsimonious predictors.

Fishbein (1982) claims researchers have shown strong relationships between smoking intentions and smoking behaviors. The majority of people who say they will not smoke, do not, and those that say they will smoke, do. Also, he found considerable evidence supporting the argument that personalized beliefs and attitudes influence the formation of behavioral intentions. Determining behavioral intent, according to Fishbein (1982), has a constraint; the specification of a time period when asking about intention is crucial. It is an often overlooked factor in many attempts to predict behavior from intention. Researchers can make more accurate predictions if they shorten the interval between measuring intention and observing the behavior (Fishbein, 1982).

Habit

Relatively heavy smokers (those who smoke an average of 26.6 cigarettes per day) may be less likely to join cessation-treatment programs (Sussman et al., 1989). These same authors suggest that the level of one's use of cigarettes throughout the day (which may reflect nicotine dependence) may influence one's self-efficacy about being able to complete treatment and one's initial decision about joining treatment. Ockene et al., (1982) claim that having few cigarettes smoked upon entry into their program was among six factors that when combined demonstrated the likelihood that the individual could stop and maintain cessation.

In a study of 1,501 smokers, cigarette consumption, regularity of smoking, type of cigarette, and inhalation were among the factors studied. At about 20 cigarettes daily, smoking becomes a regular event, with smokers inhaling "a lot" or "a fair amount." The heavier smokers were less confident in their ability to change permanently to mild cigarettes (Russell et al., 1980). More relevant to the present study is the evidence showing that persons smoking more than 10 cigarettes per day are less likely to quit (Gordon, Kannel, and Dawber, 1975). In the Weinberger et al., 1981 study of 120 respondents, ex-smokers had smoked for a shorter period of time when compared with the moderate smoker and smoker groups.

Habit may be related to a person's belief that he or she is capable of beginning a program or even quitting smoking. Ockene et al., (1982) predicted with 81% accuracy which smokers would have problems with smoking cessation. Although habit is a factor, its relative weight (predictive value as a sole factor) is unknown. In this study the problem smokers were the least personally secure. Personal security is a subjective evaluation of oneself as successful, satisfied, and confident with respect to the carrying out of one's purposes in past, present, and future situations and group relations. In addition, problem smokers attended fewer group sessions, had the least positive smoking environments, and smoked the most cigarettes at entry into the study.

Attitude and Subjective Norm

According to Fishbein (1982) attitude toward a behavior (the individual's positive or negative evaluation of performing a behavior) and the subjective norm (the person's perception of the social pressures put on him or her to perform or not perform a behavior) are the determinants of intentions. Generally speaking, people will intend to perform a behavior when they evaluate it positively and when they believe that important others think they should perform it.

According to Ajzen and Fishbein (1980), the first step in predicting and understanding behavioral intention is to obtain a measure of the person's attitude toward his or her performance of the behavior in question. However, the measure of attitude must correspond specifically to the measure of intention. Regarding measuring attitude, Osgood, Suci, and Tannenbaum (1957) state that attitudes can be ascribed to a basic bipolar continuum with a neutral or zero reference point and have both direction and intensity. The "characterization of attitude as a learned implicit process, which is potentially bipolar, varies in its intensity, and mediates evaluative behavior, suggests that attitude is part ...of the internal mediational activity that operates between most stimulus and response patterns" (p. 190).

Social Norms

A smoker whose significant other also smokes would be less likely to break group norms by joining a cessation program (Sussman et al., 1989). Based on literature on group dynamics, Foss (1973) noted the futility of attempting to change a person's behavior without taking into account the groups of which he or she is a member. If a smoker resides in a social group of smokers, it is rather doubtful he or she can be induced to stop by anything less than other equally strong social influence pressures "which can no doubt be had by switching social groups" (Foss, 1973, p. 284). A change in workplace because of the presence of smokers is not an issue to be researched in the present study. More important is viewing the social norm of the workplace as a factor in an individual's decision to begin a smoking-cessation program.

The modern work setting is a large part of one's life and locus of self-esteem (Kaplan, Cassel, and Gore, 1977). The work environment (setting) can be termed the social network. Schaefer, Coyne, and Lazarus (1981) define social network as a "specific set of linkages among a defined set of persons" (p. 384), or the set of relationships a person has. The network can be described in terms of its composition and structure (the number of people involved and the number who know each other) or by the content of particular relationships (friendship vs. kinship). Each particular network determines its norms, and perhaps the norms of the environment may be the crucial components that help determine desire to begin a smoking-cessation program. Another reason for obtaining social network measures is, they encompass psychological processes that may have negative consequences. Negative processes include the stressful demands made by others, the constraints others exercise over one's choices, and the disappointments often inherent in such relationships (when help is needed but not provided) (Schaefer, Coyne, and Lazarus, 1981).

Many researchers have studied the social network in the context of smoking cessation, and for the most part the results are consistent. Giannetti, Reynolds, and Rihn (1985) found that it was not the number of persons in the participant's social network that accounted for the differences between smokers and ex-smokers. Instead, it was the degree to which individuals in the network directly and frequently encouraged cessation or conversely tolerated smoking. Giannetti, Reynolds, and Rihn (1985) also cite studies indicating that social networks, which discourage smoking have been associated with successful cessation. Along the same lines, a workplace norm defining quitting smoking as "deviant" is likely to impede efforts to quit smoking. Moreover, persons receiving considerable discouragement from their co-workers have less confidence in their ability to quit (Sorensen, Pechacek, and Pallonen, 1986).

Other findings concern the characteristics of individuals having to deal with the smoking norm in their network. "Individuals who objected to others smoking around them and who used or requested nonsmoking areas in public accommodations were more likely to be nonsmokers a year following cessation. . ." (Horowitz, Hindi-Alexander, and Wagner, 1985, p. 37). According to Eisinger (1971) who studied psychosocial predictors of smoking recidivism, one environmental factor related to successful abstinence was the smoking behavior of the 20 people whom the participant knew best. Finally, results of a five-year follow-up of a smoking withdrawal clinic population showed that smokers were more likely to smoke on the job. In addition, the mother, father, friends, and co-workers of nonsmokers were more likely not to be smoking (West et al., 1977).

Self-efficacy

Self-efficacy is the individual's belief that he or she has the skills or abilities necessary to perform the behaviors that a situation demands to produce the desired outcome (Coelho, 1985). Researchers in the area of smoking-cessation and self-efficacy have found this factor to have predictive use. According to Yates and Thain (1985), self-efficacy measures may be used to identify individuals at high risk for relapse after voluntarily quitting smoking. However, more important, self-efficacy may indicate that remedial measures need to be applied before the decision to quit (which would reduce the probability of relapse). Also, in a study of smokers who attended an orientation to a smoking-cessation program, researchers found that nonjoiners had lower self-efficacy than treatment joiners (Brod and Hall, 1984).

Predictive factors are of practical significance, because they can be modified and brought under self-control with or without professional intervention (Prochaska et al., 1985). According to these researchers, self-efficacy and the smoking decision can affect whether people take action on their smoking, achieve cessation, maintain their change, or relapse. Prochaska et al., (1985) claim self-efficacy represents the subject's level of confidence he or she can resist smoking across a number of tempting situations. This factor contributed strongly in the prediction of changes in the smoking status of participants. Self-efficacy was a decisive factor both for individual's changing from contemplation (deciding whether to quit or not), to action (attempting to quit), and from action to maintenance.

Barriers

Kirscht and Rosenstock (1982) term barriers those factors associated with low rates of compliance in medical regimens. Among those listed in the study were the complexity, duration, and amount of change involved in the regimen itself; inconveniences associated with the question of clinics; inadequate supervision by professionals; and patient dissatisfaction. According to Kirscht and Rosenstock, action is thought to be more likely where it is seen as efficacious and possible at a tolerable cost. Knowing that a person perceives no barriers to his or her action indicates the person is even more likely to carry out the intention. Since a variety of forces in the individual's situation can serve as barriers to action, or as in this case barriers to intention, all perceived impediments to action should be accounted for.

Vertinsky and Auman (1988) shed additional light on the meaning and relevance of barriers. They wrote "a kind of cost-benefit analysis occurs whereby individuals weigh the desired action's effectiveness against their perceptions that it may be expensive, risky, unhealthy, inconvenient, and/or time consuming," (p. 16). Barriers to smoking cessation also can be termed reasons to continue smoking and include the following:

* the addiction to nicotine;
* social mores (acceptance of smoking behavior);
* the belief that negative consequences are delayed and probable;
* strength of the smoking habit (each puff reinforces continuance);
* encouragement to smoke by other smokers, advertisers, friends, and co-workers;
* fear of weight gain (Klesges, Cigrang, and Glasgow, 1987).

These "disadvantages to having worksite programs" are also barriers to joining. Furthermore, participating in a worksite smoking-cessation program, say Vertinsky and Auman (1988), may interfere with work activities or be tolerated, but not supported, by a supervisor or other co-worker. In addition, meetings may be held at inconvenient times (e.g., employees may have to give up other valued activities or temporarily reduce their productivity to attend).

Martin (1987) listed five frequently heard "obstacles" raised by persons who consider smoking cessation: (1) I'm afraid I'll gain weight; (2) It's my health -- don't tell me what to do with it; (3) I can quit anytime I want to -- right now I just don't want to; (4) I don't smoke that much; and (5) Smoking relieves my stress and that's good (p. 59).

Social Support

Across a variety of methods and physical disorders, there is consistent evidence that naturally occurring support is beneficial (Wallston et al., 1983). The literature is replete with differing definitions of, uses for, and definitive and nondefinitive results of social support. Two primary dimensions of social support are quantitative versus qualitative aspects, as well as instrumental versus expressive aspects. The former can be operationalized in terms of "amount" measures, such as the number of people one interacts with, the frequency of contact with specific types of others, and the frequency of contact among those others; or "goodness" measures, such as perceptions or judgments about the adequacy of interpersonal contacts. The latter can be operationalized as providing material aid and information versus serving as confidant and providing acceptance and understanding (Wallston et al., 1983).

Schaefer, Coyne, and Lazarus (1981) defined social support as an appraisal of whether and to what extent an interaction, pattern of interaction, or relationship is helpful. The three types of social support include emotional, tangible, and informational. According to these researchers, each has specific characteristics. The types of support and the characteristics relevant to the present study include emotional support - intimacy and attachment, reassurance and being able to confide in and rely on another; tangible support - direct aid or services; and informational support - information, advice, and feedback. Informational support in the form of feedback can help a person maintain a social identity and a sense of social integration, according to Schaefer, Coyne, and Lazarus (1981). However, "tangible and informational support also may serve as an emotional support function, as when they signal caring and are not viewed as resulting from obligation" (p. 385).

Finally, Westman, Eden, and Shirom (1985) cite a concurring definition of social support - a flow of emotional concern, instrumental aid, information and/or appraisal among individuals. This consensus on the concept of social support validates the measure and helps ascertain whether social support is a factor worthy of study.

It may appear that the measures of social norms (defined earlier) and social support overlap in some instances; however, there is a clear distinction. To ascertain whether one or both factors determine the likelihood that a smoker would begin a cessation program, both a structural measure (social norms) and an evaluative measure (social support) are essential. The former is a measure of the prevalence of smoking and level of acceptance. The latter is a subjective measure of encouragement or discouragement of smoking.

Although Coppotelli and Orleans (1985) cite studies showing that naturally occurring social support from significant others contributes to cessation maintenance in both retrospective and prospective studies, findings of social support before a program, in relation to the workplace, are not particularly abundant. However, findings relating other environments and non-co-workers are relevant. Results of a study of psychosocial mediators of abstinence, relapse, and continued smoking showed that social support, particularly that of spouse and friends, was confirmed to be an important factor differentiating the quitters from those that relapsed at one-year follow-up. "Ex-smokers perceived significantly greater social support at follow-up than at pretreatment from all sources measured" (Horowitz, Hindi-Alexander, and Wagner, 1985, p. 37).

Janis and Hoffman (1970) claim that for a person undergoing self-imposed deprivations such as quitting smoking, the availability of a buddy who can be contacted whenever social support is needed may help him or her maintain the appropriate attitudes and to reduce anxiety so that he or she is better able to keep the commitment. In addition, "...continued self-regulatory behavior requires social support; like any other behavior, it will extinguish in the absence of the appropriate reinforcement" (Wilson and Brownell, 1980, p. 76).

Specific studies of social support (although not work related) indicated the following. Partner facilitation was the most powerful predictor of abstinence and recidivism, accurately discriminating between the two in 85% of 125 newly abstinent married women (Coppotelli and Orleans, 1985). Others also confirmed the importance of social support for the discontinuance of smoking.   In a retrospective analysis of hospitalized cardiovascular patients, researchers found informal social support for cessation was the factor that explained the greatest difference between smokers and ex-smokers (Giannetti, Reynolds, and Rihn, 1985).

Of the few studies that specifically relate the workplace with social support, Westman, Eden, and Shirom (1985) looked at the conditioning effects of peer support as it related to job stress, smoking, and cessation.   They reported that persons having low support smoked significantly more than those who had high support.   More important, however, they claim that social support mediated the effect of job stress on the ability to quit smoking.   "A literature review on smoking yielded that people who engage in socially supportive work activities smoke, not so much to relieve tension but as a social habit perhaps reinforced by group norms..." (Westman, Eden, and Shirom, 1985, p. 642).

MODEL AND APPROACH

The Feldman model (Figure 1), comprised of the variables behavioral intent, habit, attitude, subjective norm, self-efficacy, barriers, and social support, was derived from the Wallston and Wallston (1984) unified social psychological model of health behavior.   According to Quinn (1987), the original health behavior model is based on the relationship that behavior = behavioral interest + habit + facilitating conditions.   Feldman and Mayhew's (1984) used the model by applying it to nutritional behaviors. They found that ten variables contributed to explaining meat and salt consumption, but the Wallston and Wallston (1984) model was unwieldy because of the number and complexity of the variables.

The Feldman model, the result of maintaining the best predictors of behavior and adding self-efficacy and social support, was then tested by Quinn (1987).   This model "is a two-stage model: behavior is a function of habit, intention, and self-efficacy; at the next stage of the model, intention is a function of attitude and subjective norm; and self-efficacy is a function of social support and perceived barriers," (Quinn, 1987, p. 11).   The study found all of the variables contributed to the predictions of both breast feeding and calcium intake. Specifically, attitude and subjective norm predicted behavioral intent to breast feed (53% of variance explained) and calcium intake (60% of variance explained).

The literature supports both the rationale for the present study and the approach used to collect the data. Quinn's (1987) testing of the Feldman model involved using semantic differential scales to examine habit, attitudes, intent, subjective norm, self-efficacy, perceived barriers, and social support and yielded reliability measures from .796 to .911. The questionnaire used in her study and a smoking-cessation survey developed by Feldman, Forster, and Bentley (1988) were used as models.

Although few in number, studies that have compared joiners to nonjoiners have looked at habit and social norm. For example, smoking behavior and history items were requested by Sussman et al., (1989). Respondents indicated number of cigarettes smoked the day before, number of cigarettes usually smoked in one day, number of years smoking, and number and duration of quitting attempts. The smoking environment items included whether the smokers' spouse, children, or anyone else the respondents lived with, and co-workers smoked cigarettes.

Summary

Although demographic factors as a rule are not open to change, psychosocial ones are. For this reason, those factors that can be manipulated, or (at least to some degree) controlled by the individual should be studied. Ockene et al., (1981) claimed that psychosocial assets were essential for success in quitting smoking. These assets are (1) a perception of oneself as competent and personally secure, (2) a belief in one's ability to control what happens to oneself, and (3) the availability of "significant others" for emotional support. Similarly, we expected the measures of general behavioral intent, habit, attitude, subjective norm, social norms, self-efficacy, barriers, and social support to predict who intends to join a specific worksite smoking-cessation program.

METHOD

Subjects

The population was comprised of Department of Labor (DOL) employees of the Washington metropolitan area. All DOL employees (6,606) were sent questionnaires through interoffice mail to obtain a sample of smokers.

Instrument

To enhance the "feeling of anonymity" and contain costs, we chose a written questionnaire as the mode of data collection. The questionnaire was designed to obtain the measures of eight factors (predictive variables, which included a measure of general behavioral intent) to judge their effect on the criterion variable-intention to join the next available worksite smoking-cessation program. The questionnaire was pretested on 10 DOL employees.

Procedure

After pretesting the questionnaire and making minor adjustments, it was given to the Assistant Secretary for Administration and Management at DOL.   He wrote a memorandum to the employees requesting their participation, and submitted it to the department's print shop to be printed and disseminated.

Item 1 on the questionnaire was a screening device: potential respondents indicated whether or not they were cigarette smokers and only smokers were asked to continue to the next page.

Items 2-7 were designed to obtain a measure of habit. Specifically, two items to determine the subject's degree of smoking habit, three items to determine past joining behavior, and one to determine if the person had ever stopped smoking as a result of a program.

Items 8-11 were designed to obtain a measure of social norms to determine whether none, some, half, most, or all of the subject's co-workers and friends smoke. The lower the scores, the more smoking was the norm. The respondent also was asked for the number of people he or she resides with and how many of those individuals smoke.

Items 12-18 measured attitude. They were used to determine if the subject was favorably disposed toward not smoking (three items) and joining a smoking cessation program (four items). On semantic differential scales of 1 to 7 for each item, the lower the score, the more favorably disposed the respondent was to not smoking and joining a program. The measure of subjective norm was comprised of four items (19-22). The purpose was to determine to what degree subjects think their co-workers, spouses/partners, and friends think they should join a smoking-cessation program. The lower the score, on a scale of 1 (agree) to 7 (disagree), the more the subject believed these significant others were favorably disposed.

The social support measure was comprised of items 23-26. Each respondent indicated if he or she received encouragement to join a smoking cessation program. Scores ranged from 1 (often) to 4 (never); the lower the score, the more supportive the co-workers, spouse/partner, friends, and family members.

Items 27-31 were used to indicate the subject's confidence (self-efficacy) in his or her ability to find and join a smoking-cessation program. Scores ranged from 1 (confident) to 7 (not confident); the lower the score, the more certain the individual was of his or her ability.

Items 32-37 enabled the subject to indicate to what extent barriers - cost, inconvenience, embarrassment, time, or work - would prevent him or her from joining a smoking cessation program. Respondents were given a space to specify an unlisted barrier. For each item, scores ranged from 1 (not prevent me) to 7 (prevent me). The higher the score, the more the subject perceived the barrier as a stumbling block.

Items 38-42 were designed to elicit one of two measures of behavioral intent. These items correspond to the degree of intent to join a program, complete a program, or stop smoking. Based on semantic differential scales of 1 to 7 for each item, the lower the score, the more the respondent intended to join a program, complete a program, or stop smoking.

Additional variables were item 43, a self-evaluation (on a scale of 1 (smoker) to 7 (ex-smoker) of how close a respondent believes he or she is to becoming a smoker or ex-smoker; items 44-48 were used to elicit data that will be useful for smoking-cessation program planners; and items 49-53 were needed to obtain the demographic data. The last page of the questionnaire requested that the respondent should only return this page if he or she would like to join the next smoking-cessation program. It was a measure of specific intention.

RESULTS

Over the course of three weeks, 689 respondents (10.42%) returned questionnaires to a worksite location (the Local 12, American Federation of Government Employees office). Of all the questionnaires returned, 486 were nonsmokers (70.53%) and 203 were smokers (29.46%). [The percentage of smokers who responded is consistent with the result of an unpublished DOL survey, which found that roughly 25% of its employees are smokers.] Of the 203 smokers, 35 were excluded because one or more questionnaire pages were missing. This left a sample of 168 usable questionnaires (24.38%). Forty respondents (23.8%) indicated they wanted to join the next available worksite program.

Two of the factors under study were eliminated from consideration (social norms and self-efficacy) or modified (habit, attitude, barriers, and ethnicity) during the analysis of data. The rationale for each elimination or modification follows. First, an attempt was made to combine questionnaire items to form scales. The social norm measure was eliminated because the items did not form a reliable scale (alpha=.36, and individually the items were not correlated with either measure of behavioral intent (the correlations ranged from -.04 to .17).

Although the measure of self-efficacy formed a reliable scale, because of the way the instructions were worded (respondents were instructed to skip items 27-31 if they were not considering a stop-smoking program), more than half of the respondents skipped the section on the questionnaire. Such a small number of cases (76) would have adversely affected the analysis of the other variables.

Four modifications were made. On the habit measure, five of the original components were dropped; only the number of smoking-cessation programs previously joined was used. Since intention to join is the criterion variable, the number of previous programs joined is the logical and appropriate measure of habit (past behavior).

The attitude measure was modified as well. One item of the scale was dropped. According to Osgood, May, and Miron (1975), when used on a semantic differential scale, the qualifiers valuable-worthless, useful-usefulness, and wise-foolish are evaluative judgments. Easy-difficult, however, is a judgment of potency and is neither empirically nor theoretically a measure of the same construct. In other words, using the first three sets of qualifiers, respondents evaluated joining the program. Using the potency judgment, they were in fact rating their ability to join a program. Hence, one item was dropped.

Originally the barriers measure was comprised of six items; however, the sixth was dropped. Five barriers were listed, respondents were asked to list the sixth. Given the wide variety of responses, classification under major headings was not possible. The final modification involved collapsing data on ethnicity (Table 1) to two categories: Black and White.

Findings

Reliability measures of each of the scales were obtained. Alpha reliability for the usable scales ranged from .73 to .90. The alpha reliability for the social norms scale was .36 (Table 2). Next, correlation coefficients were obtained; seven of the original predictor variables are shown in Table 3.

Six scales (habit, attitude, subjective norm, social support, barriers, and general behavioral intent) and three demographic variables were analyzed to determine the predictors of intention to join a worksite smoking-cessation program.

First, a multivariate test of significance of the combined six predictor variables and a demographic variable (G.S. level) was conducted (Hotellings T^2=0.27, F[7,111]=4.23, p<.000). The univariate tests indicated no variable was significant except for general behavioral intent. The results show that the greater the general intention to join a program, the greater the specific intention to join (F[1,117]=19.22, p<.000). In addition, the lower the G.S. level, the greater the specific intention to join (F[1,117]=7.05, p<.009) (Table 4). Differences between intenders (respondents who intend to join the next available worksite cessation program) and nonintenders are listed in Table 5.

Chi-square values were obtained for the relationship between intention to join and demographic variables. Twenty-two Black employees (38.6%) and 12 White employees (12.1%) indicated they wanted to join the next available worksite smoking-cessation program (Chi-square=14.88, df=1; p<.0001). The second significant finding using the Chi-square statistic involved union membership (Chi-square=9.35, df=1; p<.002). Of the 39 intenders who indicated membership status, 19 (39.6%) were union members. Of those not intending to join, 82.8% were not union members.

Multiple regression was used to determine the predictability of specific behavioral intent. The predictor variables were general behavioral intent, habit, attitude, subjective norm, social support, barriers, ethnicity, G.S. level, and union membership (Table 6). Using the enter method of multiple regression, each variable was evaluated for its contribution to the model for predicting specific behavioral intent. The amount of variance explained was 23.6%. The variables with the greatest contribution were general behavioral intent and ethnicity: general intent explained 13% and ethnicity explained 8.1%. Individuals who expressed a greater (general) intention to join a program were more likely to join the specified program. Also, Black employees expressed greater intention to join than White employees.

These values were verified using the stepwise method of multiple regression. Together the two variables (general intent and ethnicity) explained 21.1% of the variance, and all other variables were dropped from the equation for lack of significance.

Using both the enter and stepwise methods of multiple regression with general behavioral intent as the criterion variable, the set of variables explained 35.1% of the variance. Subjective norm, habit, and attitude were the greatest contributors (R^2=33.8; F=18.56; p<.0000) (Table 7).

It is not a surprise that generalized intention is the best predictor of intention to join a specific worksite program. However, why should more Black employees want to join a worksite program, and why are the best predictors for the general and specific measures different? The following discussion will focus on the factors that may be responsible for these findings.

In designing this study we were prepared for a difference in the measures of behavioral intent. Clearly a difference exists between a general intention to do something and a specified intention. Perhaps the degree of specificity or commitment is responsible for the other factors having no significant predictive value for intending to join the specified program.

Hallett and Sutton (1987) found that only 61% of those who volunteered to participate in a program attended a session. Also, Lowe, Windsor, and Post (1987) show how the greater the commitment, the fewer the committed. One hundred and nineteen smokers stated on a questionnaire that they would be interested in participating in a quit-smoking program. Two groups were formed: a randomized sample of forty-six individuals (Group 1) were sent letters of invitation and none responded. Group 2 was a randomized sample of forty-four. Thirty-seven of them received the invitation in a personal phone call. Of that thirty-seven, only nineteen made appointments and seven kept them (Lowe, Windsor, and Post, 1987).

To account for the discrepancy in the measures of behavioral intention in the present study, several points must be considered: (1) the noncomparable formats of the primary and secondary measures, and (2) the dissimilarity of the two measures. On the first measure of behavioral intent, respondents indicated on a scale of 1 (agree) to 7 (disagree), the extent to which they intended to join a stop-smoking program within 1 year, complete a stop-smoking program within 1 year, join a stop-smoking program in 3 months, stop smoking, and join a stop-smoking program at work. Each statement began with "I intend to. . . ." The second measure, however, was much more specific - "I want to join the next Stop-Smoking Program." What was originally conceived as a small difference between general intention (what a respondent actually intended to do) and commitment or specific intention (what a respondent actually wants to do) is really a major difference in terms of how each respondent perceived and responded to the items.

Given the moderate ability of this model to predict specific intention, why then the importance of demographic variables and lack of importance of other factors? Although it is not clear why more Blacks than Whites would want to join a worksite smoking-cessation program, the following should be considered. What may appear to be an ethnic difference, may in fact be a socioeconomic difference. Data on smokers in the general population (Koop, 1985) indicate the claimed ethnic difference regarding smoking behavior appears to be more of a working class difference (Table 8). Note that as occupational level decreases, the percentage of smokers increases (except for Black females).

In the present study the ethnic factor may be comprised of hidden characteristics such as a class difference (reflected in G.S. level), union membership, and a differential response rate. When ethnicity and G.S. level are examined, one finds that there are more Black than White employees in the lower grade levels. Here too, ethnicity masks socioeconomic and demographic factors.

Nineteen of 35 joiners indicated their grade levels (54.3%) and 31 of the 51 Black employees who indicated their grade levels (60.8%) were G.S. level 7 or less (Table 9).

The Chi-square value was obtained for the relationship between ethnicity and union membership (Chi-square=24.46, p<.0000). Of the 154 respondents who indicated their ethnicity and status of union membership, 52.7% of Blacks belonged to the union versus 15.2% of Whites. It also should be noted that the application form showed the next program was co-sponsored by the union. Perhaps more union members (hence more Black employees) were motivated to participate.

One final consideration: 50% of the DOL workforce is Black; however, only one-third of the respondents are Black. And, as was mentioned previously, the range of G.S. levels for sample respondents was 3 to 16. The mean G.S. level for respondents, those intending to join, and nonintenders was 10.5, 9.0, and 11.0, respectively. So respondents tended to be of high G.S. level (a possible indicator of a differential response rate) with White respondents having higher G.S. level and being nonintenders.

There is no clear-cut answer why more Blacks than Whites would be interested in joining a worksite program. However, what is clear is that the Black intenders do not represent Black DOL employees. Black employees who took the time to fill out and return the questionnaire were of relatively high G.S. levels and were more interested in joining. (It also should be noted that Rost et al., [1987] found nonmanagement employees were more likely to participate in worksite health promotion programs.)

The results of this study show that the predictive value of the Feldman model rests with the ability to predict general intention. General intention is the predictor of specific intention. The variables habit, attitude, subjective norm, social support, barriers, general behavioral intent, and G.S. level can distinguish between those intending and not intending to join a worksite smoking-cessation program.

SUMMARY AND CONCLUSIONS

The number of employees who smoke and the toll their smoking takes on their employers is well documented. And although researchers of smoking cessation are beginning to look at the unique contribution of the workplace as another area in the struggle against smoking, little research has addressed which factors predict who joins smoking-cessation programs, much less who intends to join.

The purpose of this study was to determine to what extent social support, social norms, habit, self-efficacy, attitude, subjective norm, barriers, and a general measure of behavioral intent predict which smokers intend to join a specific worksite smoking-cessation program. Forty of the 168 respondents (23.8%) indicated they wanted to join the next available worksite program.

General intention was the only variable able to significantly differentiate between those intending and not intending to join a specific program (p<.05; F=.000). For those intending to join the next available worksite smoking-cessation program, the means for attitude (toward joining a program), subjective norm (what significant others think), social support, and habit (the number of programs ever joined) had more positive values, whereas the mean for perceived barriers did not.

A set of eight factors (the Feldman modification of the Wallston and Wallston [1984] social psychological model of health behavior [Quinn, 1987]) was shown to be a valid predictor of general behavioral intent. Subjective norm, attitude, and habit were the greatest contributors, and the set explained 35.1% of the variance. Generalized intention was the best predictor along with ethnicity of who intends to join a worksite smoking-cessation program. Together they explained 21.1% of the variance. A different combination of the variables (habit, attitude, subjective norm, social support, barriers, general behavioral intent, and G.S. level) were found to distinguish between those intending and not intending to join a worksite smoking-cessation program (Hottellings $T^2=0.27$, $F[7,111]=4.23$, $p<.000$).

In spite of the significance level of the finding on ethnicity, the factor ethnicity should not be regarded as a true predictor based on a difference between Black and White employees. Hidden within this factor are characteristics such as class discrepancy, union membership, and a differential response rate. Herein lie the implications of these findings: worksite smoking-cessation programs appeal more to those of comparatively lower work levels, and the program's sponsor may affect participation. That is, the involvement of and sponsorship by unions may increase the participation of union members.

Acknowledgement

The authors wish to thank the U.S. Department of Labor and the American Federation of Government Employees, Local 12, for their support in conducting this study.

REFERENCES

Ajzen, I. & Fishbein, M. (1980). *Understanding attitudes and predicting social behavior.* Englewood Cliffs, New Jersey: Prentice Hall.

Biener, L., Carey, M., McAnulty, D., Follick, M. & Abrams, P.B. (1987). *Nonparticipants in worksite smoking cessation programs.* Presented at the Society of Behavioral Medicine, March, Washington.

Brod, M.I. & Hall, S.M. (1984). Joiners and non-joiners in smoking treatment: A comparison of psychosocial variables. *Addictive Behaviors, 9,* (2), 217-221.

Coelho, R.J. (1985). *Quitting smoking: A psychological experiment using community research.* VIII/5. New York: Peter Lang.

Coppotelli, C.H. & Orleans, C.T. (1985). Partner support and other determinants of smoking cessation maintenance among women. *Journal of Consulting and Clinical Psychology, 53,* (4), 455-460.

Eisinger, R.A. (1971). Psychosocial predictors of smoking recidivism. *Journal of Health and Social Behavior,* (12), 355-362.

Feldman, R.H.L. & Mayhew, P.C. (1984). Predicting nutrition behavior: The utilization of a social psychological model of health behavior. *Basic and Applied Social Psychology, 5,* (3), 183-195.

Feldman, R.H.L., Forster, J. & Bentley, M.K. (1988). *Psychosocial factors in a union-based worksite smoking cessation study.* Paper presented at the American Public Health Association meeting, Boston, Massachusetts.

Fishbein, M. (1982).   Social psychological analysis of smoking behavior.   In *Social psychology and behavioral medicine,* J.R. Eiser (Ed.).   New York: John Wiley.

Foss, R. (1973).   Personality, social influence, and cigarette smoking. *Journal of Health and Social Behavior, 14,* (9), 279-286.

Giannetti, V.J., Reynolds, J., & Rihn, T. (1985).   Factors which differentiate   smokers   from   ex-smokers   among cardiovascular patients: A discriminant analysis. *Social Science and Medicine, 20,* (2), 241-245.

Glasgow, R.E., Klesges, R.C. & Klesges, L.M. (1987). *Predicting participation and outcome in worksite smoking control.* Presented   at   the   Society   of   Behavioral   Medicine, Washington, D.C.

Gordon, T., Kannel, W.B., Dawber, T.R., et al., (1975).   Changes associated   with   quitting   cigarette   smoking: The Framingham Study. *American Heart Journal, 90,* 322-328.

Hallett, R. & Sutton, S.R. (1987).   Predicting participation and outcome in four workplace smoking intervention programs. *Health Education Research, 2,* (3), 257-266.

Horowitz, M.B., Hindi-Alexander, M. & Wagner, T. (1985). Psychosocial   mediators   of   abstinence,   relapse,   and continued smoking: A one-year follow-up on a minimal intervention. *Addictive Behaviors, 10,* 29-39.

Janis, I.L. & Hoffman, D. (1970).   Facilitating effects of daily contact between partners who make a decision to cut down on smoking. *Journal of Personality and Social Psychology, 17,* (1), 25-35.

Kaplan, B.H., Cassell, J.C. & Gore, S. (1977). Social support and health. *Medical Care, 15,* (5), 47-58.

Kirscht, J.P. & Rosenstock, I.M. (1982). Patients' problems in following recommendations of health experts. In *Health psychology -- A handbook,* G.C. Stone et al. (Eds.) San Francisco, California: Jossey-Bass.

Klesges, R.C., Cigrang, J. & Glasgow, R.E. (1987). Worksite smoking modification programs: A state-of-the-art review and directions for future research. *Current Psychological Research & Reviews, 6,* (1), 26-56.

Koop, C.E. (1985). *The health consequences of smoking: A report of the surgeon general.* U.S. Government Printing Office: Washington, D.C.

Lowe, J.B., Windsor, R.A. & Post, K.L. (1987). Effectiveness of impersonal versus interpersonal methods to recruit employees into a worksite quit smoking program. *Addictive Behaviors, 12,* (3), 281-284.

Martin, R.S. (1987). The anatomy of motivation: Can we and will we change? *Family and Community Health, 10,* (3), 57-60.

Ockene, J.K., Benfari, R.C., Nuttall, R.L., Hurwitz, I. & Ockene, I.S. (1981). A psychosocial model of smoking cessation and maintenance cessation. *Preventive Medicine, 10,* 623-638.

Ockene, J.K. et al., (1982). Relationship of psychosocial factors to smoking behavior change in an intervention program. *Preventive Medicine, 11,* 13-28.

Osgood, C.E., Suci, G.J. & Tannenbaum, P.H. (1957). *The measurement of meaning.* University of Illinois Press: Chicago.

Osgood, C.E., May, W.H. & Miron, M.S. (1975). *Cross cultural universals of affective meanings.* University of Illinois Press: Chicago.

Prochaska, J.O., DiClemente, C.C., Velicer, S. & Norcross, J.C. (1985). Predicting change in smoking status for self-changers. *Addictive Behaviors, 10,* 395-406.

Quinn, E.B. (1987). *Psychosocial determinants of breast feeding and the intake of dietary calcium of pregnancy,* Doctoral dissertation, University of Maryland, College Park.

Rost, K., Barzilai, B., Schechtman, K. & Fisher, E.B. (1987). *Predictors of participation in worksite health promotion programs: Are we preaching to the converted?* Presented at the Society of Behavioral Medicine, Washington, D.C.

Russell, M.A.H. et al., (1980). Smoking habits of men and women. *British Medical Journal, 5,* (July), 17-20.

Schaefer, C., Coyne, J.C. & Lazarus, R.S. (1981). The health-related functions of social support. *Journal of Behavioral Medicine, 4,* (4), 381-405.

Sorensen, G., Pechacek, T. & Pallonen, U. (1986). Occupational and worksite norms and attitudes about smoking cessation. *American Journal of Public Health, 76,* (5), 544-549.

Sussman, S., Whitney-Saltiel, D.A., Budd, R.J. et al., (1989). Joiners and non-joiners in worksite smoking treatment: Pretreatment smoking, smoking by significant others, and expectation to quit as predictors. *Addictive Behaviors, 14,* 113-119.

Vertinsky, P. & Auman, J.T. (1988). Elderly women's barriers to exercise. Part I: Perceived Risks. *Health Values, 12,* (4), 13-24.

Wallston, B.S., Alagna, S.W., Devellis, B.M. & Devellis, R.F. (1983).   Social support and physical health.   *Health Psychology, 2,* (4), 367-391.

Wallston, B.S. & Wallston, K.A. (1984).   Social psychological models of health behavior: An examination and integration. In *Handbook of psychology and health,* Vol. IV, edited by A. Baum et al. Hillsdale, N.J.:   Lawrence Erlbaum Associates.

Westman, M., Eden, D. & Shirom, A. (1985).   Job stress, cigarette smoking and cessation: The conditioning effects of peer support. *Social Science and Medicine, 20,* (6), 637-644.

Wilson, G.T. & Brownell, K.D. (1980).   Behavior therapy for obesity: An evaluation of treatment outcome. *Advances in Behavior Research and Therapy, 3,* 79-86.

Weinberger, M., Greene, J.Y., Mamlin, J.J. & Jerin, J.J. (1981). Health beliefs and smoking behavior. *American Journal of Public Health, 71,* (11), 1253-1255.

Yates, A.J. & Thain, J. (1985).   Self-efficacy as a predictor of relapse following voluntary cessation of smoking. *Addictive behaviors, 10,* (3), 291-298.

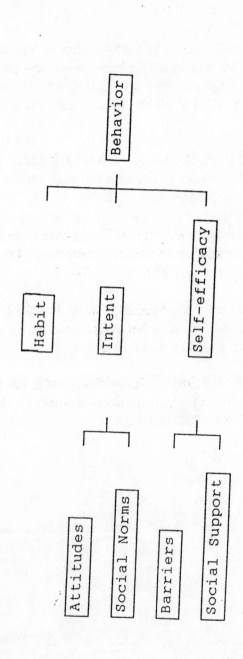

Figure 1. Unified social psychological model of health behavior of Wallston and Wallston, modified by Feldman (Source: Quinn, 1987).

Table 1

Distribution of Sample by Demographics

Gender	Male		Female		N/A	
Frequency	73		91		4	
% of sample	43.5		44.5		2.4	

Age	20-30	30-40	40-50	50-60	>60	N/A
Frequency	26	54	57	23	5	3
% of sample	15.5	32.1	33.9	13.7	3.0	1.8

Ethnicity	Black	White	Hispanic	Other	N/A
Frequency	57	99	4	3	5
% of sample	33.9	58.9	2.4	1.8	3.0

Union Member	Yes	No	N/A
Frequency	48	116	4
% of sample	28.6	69.0	2.4

Table 2

Reliability of the Scales

Scale	Number of Items	Alpha Reliability
Habit	1	--
Social Norm	3	.36
Attitude (smoking)	3	.73
Attitude (joining)	3	.88
Attitude (smoking+joining)	6	.85
Subjective norm	4	.86
Social support	3	.82
Self-efficacy	5	.88
Barriers	5	.80
General Behavioral Intent	5	.90

Table 3

Intercorrelation Matrix
of Predictors of Behavioral Intent

Variable		HJOINNO	ATJT	SBNT	SST	SEFFT	BART	INTT
ATJT	r=	-.066						
	p=	.220						
	N=	141						
SBNT	r=	-.142	.487					
	p=	.045	.000					
	N=	144	134					
SST	r=	-.229	.398	.780				
	p=	.002	.000	.000				
	N=	150	133	144				
SEFFT	r=	-.195	.104	.296	.293			
	p=	.048	.200	.007	.008			
	N=	74	67	69	69			
BART	r=	.046	-.070	-.054	-.100	.384		
	p=	.283	.203	.262	.114	.000		
	N=	156	142	144	147	76		
INTT	r=	-.197	.442	.500	.469	.677	-.079	
	p=	.007	.000	.000	.000	.000	.164	
	N=	154	141	143	146	72	155	
BINT	r=	-.081	.183	.122	.175	.051	-.120	.391
	p=	.151	.014	.070	.015	.332	.066	.000
	N=	164	145	148	153	76	160	158
	t=	-1.04	2.22	1.48	2.18	.44	-1.51	5.30

HJOINNO=habit (number of programs joined), ATJT=attitude, SBNT=subject-
ive norm, SST=social support, SEFFT=self-efficacy, BART=barriers, INTT=general
behavioral intent, BINT=specific behavioral intent.

Table 4

Univariate Tests of Variables
That Distinquish between Intending and Not
Intending To Join Worksite Cessation Programs

Variables	F	Significance
Habit	3.22	.075
Attitudes	3.00	.086
Subjective norm	1.61	.208
Social support	3.07	.082
Barriers	0.31	.578
General intent	19.22	.000
G.S. level	7.05	.009

The criterion for significance results from
applying the Bonferroni correction factor, which
indicates that .007 is the approriate level of
significance.

Table 5

Differences between Intending and Not Intending To Join
Worksite Smoking Cessation Programs

Variable	Intenders			Nonintenders			
	N	Mean	S.D.	N	Mean	S.D.	Range
Habit	38	.47	.9	126	.33	.4	0-4
Attitude	33	7.85	4.0	112	10.01	5.1	3-21
Subj. Norm	36	15.56	7.7	112	17.72	7.6	4-28
Soc. Support	35	10.51	3.8	118	11.98	3.4	4-16
Barriers	37	19.27	8.8	123	16.88	8.3	5-35
Gen. Intent	36	19.47[1]	9.8	122	27.58	7.5	5-35
G.S. Level	35	8.97	3.6	123	10.97	3.4	3-16

Significance level $p < .05$; $F = .000$. The Bonferonni correction
was used to determine the appropriate level of significance.
Note: For all variables except habit and G.S. level, the lower
the mean score, the greater the value of the variable.

Table 6

Multiple Regression Predicting Specific Behavioral Intent

Variable	Standard Reg. Coeff.	Change in R^i	Cumulative R^i	F	Sign. F
General intent	.36	.130	.130	16.62	.0001
Habit	.02	.001	.131	8.26	.0005
Attitude	-.02	.000	.131	5.47	.0015
Subjective norm	-.09	.006	.137	4.27	.0030
Social support	.13	.013	.144	3.59	.0049
Barriers	.02	.000	.144	2.97	.0101
Ethnicity	.30	.081	.225	4.36	.0003
G.S. level	.12	.010	.235	4.00	.0004
Union	.04	.001	.236	3.54	.0007

Table 7

Multiple Regression Predicting General Behavioral Intent

Variable	Standard Reg. Coeff.	Change in R^i	Cumulative R^i	F	Sign. F
Habit	-.29	.086	.086	10.42	.0016
Attitude	.42	.174	.260	19.31	.0000
Subjective norm	.32	.078	.338	18.56	.0000
Social support	.16	.010	.348	14.43	.0000
Barriers	.00	.000	.348	11.44	.0000
G.S. level	.04	.002	.351	9.52	.0000
Ethnicity	.02	.000	.351	8.09	.0000
Union	.03	.000	.351	7.03	.0000

Table 8

Breakdown of Smoking Groups

| Occupation | Black | | White | |
	Males	Females	Males	Females
Total	47.7	34.6	40.1	33.3
White collar	38.4	35.2	32.8	32.0
Blue collar	52.1	33.4	46.5	39.6
Service	48.8	33.5	47.0	38.7

Table 9

Grade Levels of Respondents

| G.S. Levels and Starting Salaries | | Number of Respondents | |
		Black	White
3-4	$12,038-13,513	4	3
5-6	$15,118-16,851	21	5
7-8	$18,726-20,739	6	3
9-10	$22,907-25,226	6	10
11-12	$27,716-33,218	9	22
13-14	$39,501-46,679	5	44
15-16	$54,907-64,397	0	11

13

CONFIRMATORY FACTOR ANALYSIS OF A MULTIDIMENSIONAL HEALTH BELIEF MODEL INVENTORY

Charles M. Cychosz
Dean F. Anderson
Thomas E. Deeter

This investigation examined the factor structure of a multidimensional inventory measuring major elements of the Health Belief Model (HBM). The HBM has been recognized as an important theoretical approach to the study of adherence to health behaviors. However, there has been a need for psychometrically sound inventories which will measure theoretical constructs of the HBM. On that basis, the 39-item inventory represented a hypothetical structure consisting of five factors. These were labeled Susceptibility (8 items), Benefits (10 items), Barriers (12 items), Social Influences (5 items) and Cues to Action (3 items). The inventory was administered to students in physical fitness (n=157) and first aid (n=178) classes. Summary statistics from confirmatory factor analysis suggest that the proposed factor structure fit these data quite well. In the hypothesized model, all factor loadings except two were over .45 and all t-values were significant ranging from 10.88 to 5.81. These results also suggest that the 39 items were appropriately grouped into the five hypothesized factors. In addition, results from the confirmatory analysis support the theoretical proposition of interactive factors within the Health Belief Model.

Regular physical activity continues to be an important aspect of contemporary health promotion and disease prevention efforts. While much of the attention has focused on reducing the risk of cardiovascular disease, exercise may also play a role in reducing perceived stress (Morgan, 1979), tension (deVries, Wisnell, Bulbulian & Moritani, 1981), and depression (Griest, Klein, Eischens, Faris, Gurman & Morgan, 1979). Additional benefits include a greater sense of self-control (Taylor, Sallis & Needle, 1985) and general well-being (Morgan, 1981). Despite this range of possible benefits, only about one-half of the population engages in any regular fitness program (Stephens, Jacobs & White, 1985). Using more rigorous definitions of fitness programs that are more clearly associated with positive physical health outcomes, only 15 to 21% of adults are found to be participating. This represents some improvement over the levels reported in the 1960s. Nonetheless, the high level of inactivity is still associated with a sizeable economic cost, both to individuals and to society (Keeler, E., Manning, W., Newhouse, J., Sloss, E., & Wasserman, J., 1989).

Concern over participation rates has also mounted as more worksite programs examine their return on investment (Iverson, Fielding, Crow & Christenson, 1985). In these worksite programs, research suggests that approximately 20% or less of all employees join programs and only about one-half of these have long-term participation (Steinhordt & Carrier, 1989). These concerns have led researchers to examine the utility of a number of theoretical models in explaining decisions about exercise. While several of these theories hold promise, the Health Belief Model (HBM; Rosenstock, 1974) is attractive for a number of reasons.

Originally developed in the 1950s, the HBM has been applied to a wide variety of compliance decisions (Rosenstock, 1974). According to the theory, the decision to comply with medical regimen is a function of several factors. First, individuals must believe that they are susceptible to the illness or to some negative consequences from non-compliance. Second, perceptions of the severity of consequences may influence one's decision regarding health practices. Perceived benefit of compliance is a third component considered in the model. Perceived barriers to action are the fourth component. Higher levels of susceptibility, severity, and benefits would predict an increase in the likelihood of compliance behavior while higher perceived barriers would be expected to decrease compliance behavior. A variety of other factors including general health motivation are also considered under personal characteristics of the individual. Finally, refinement of the model has identified cues to action, or short-term benefits, as an important link between readiness, intention, and action.

As originally conceived, the HBM also identifies possible interventions. This is particularly important from an educational perspective. A model that hypothesizes and measures non-modifiable phenomena would be a little use to professionals interested in developing more effective interventions. Also, the HBM is robust enough to accommodate model modifications as our understanding of behavior progresses. Since there is a broad range of characteristics which seem to influence decision making, it is important that the model be able to accommodate new findings. In this sense the HBM may help to unify some of the diverse theoretical perspectives concerning exercise behavior.

Disadvantages of the HBM include a history of difficulties in operationalizing constructs. The HBM has been measured by a variety of instruments, many of which were psychometrically suspect. Slenker, Price, Roberts & Jurs (1984) used an elicitation response technique in developing a questionnaire to measure the components of the HBM as they relate to decisions about running and jogging.   Slenker et al. included barriers, general health motivation, benefits, complexity, severity, susceptibility, and cues to action in the original instrument.   They administered the instrument to two groups, joggers at a race (n=124), and office workers (n=96). They found relatively high internal consistencies for most of the components: Knowledge (10 items, .30), Susceptibility (7 items, .86), Severity (7 items, .83), Benefits (11 items, .92), Barriers (9 items, .83), Complexity (3 items, .74), Support (5 items, .84), Cues to Action (3 items, .80), General Health Motivation (2 items, .57), and Locus of Control (18 items, .75). In addition, Slenker et al., (1984) found Barriers, Motivation, Benefits, Complexity, Severity, and Cues to be significant predictors of jogging behavior.

While this instrument has shown promise, use of the elicitation response technique in developing the questionnaire does not ensure that the instrument was appropriate for other populations. In fact, the elicitation response technique tends to produce items which are specific and unique to the original study population. The real value of an instrument, however, would seem to lie in its ability to measure the HBM constructs in other populations. Thus, the purpose of this investigation was to examine, using another population, whether the instrument items reflect the hypothetical structure of the Health Belief Model.

METHOD

A total of 335 undergraduate male (n=111) and female (n=224) students, enrolled in elective physical fitness (n=157) and first aid (n=178) classes, volunteered to participate. Ages ranged from 18 to 35 years (M=21.50 yrs., SD=4.65 yrs.). Responses were collected at the beginning of the semester.

Items for the Health Belief Model Inventory (HBMI) were developed with five major elements of the HBM in mind (Becker & Maimar, 1975; Becker et al., 1979). Many of the specific items were originally developed by Slenker et al., (1984) using a series of open-ended questions. These items were reviewed prior to use in this study. Some changes in wording were made in order to adapt the inventory to this population. Throughout the process of item development, a careful attempt was made to include diverse elements that might relate to adherence decisions. This resulted in a 39-item inventory representing a hypothetical structure consisting of five factors. These were labeled: Susceptibility (8 items), Benefits (10 items), Barriers (13 items), Social Influences (5 items), and Cues to Action (3 items). Each item was rated on a 7-point scale from unlikely (1) to likely (7).

This study examined how well these data fit the proposed factor structure. If data fit adequately, the HBMI would appear to be a measure to use for examining the impact of the HBM components on compliance behavior. Since the HBM suggests related factors, a confirmatory factor analysis with an oblique rotation was conducted using the LISREL VI program (Joreskog & Sorbom, 1984). In addition to testing the underlying factor structure of the hypothesized model, a comparison was made to the null model.

RESULTS

Initial analysis of the HBMI examined the internal consistency of the five hypothetical factors. Reliabilities were determined by coefficient alpha (Cronbach, 1951). Internal consistency for four of the five subscales was quite adequate with alpha coefficients varying from .89 to .84 (Table 1). Internal consistency for the Cue to Action subscale (3 item factor) was .68. Inspection of the item-to-total correlation coefficient values for four of the five subscales suggests that all of the items included within each subscale seem to contribute to that scale's total alpha coefficient. These data seem to contribute to that scale's total alpha coefficient. These data seem to suggest adequate internal consistency for at least four of the subscales of the HBMI.

Confirmatory factor analysis was conducted to determine whether the hypothetical 5-factor structure adequately described these data. A null mode, a structure in which no common factors are assumed and items are considered completely independent was also analyzed and results were compared. The summary statistics for these factor analyses are given in Table 2.

The significant Chi-square value ($X^2[692]=2104.5$, $p=.001$) clearly suggests that these data did depart from the proposed 5-factor model. However, many experts (Bentler & Bonnett, 1980; Joreskog, 1969; Joreskog & Sorbom, 1981) note that even minor discrepancies between the data and the model may yield a significant difference with large samples and a large number of degrees of freedom. Joreskog (1969) cautions against a literal interpretation of the Chi-square and specifically advocates that a ratio of Chi-square to degrees of freedom below a value of 5.0 to be considered an index of a model's acceptability when considered in conjunction with other criteria. This ratio is 3.04. In addition, the coefficient of determination 0.94, the goodness-of-fit index, 0.74, and the adjusted goodness-of-fit index, 0.70, suggest that the proposed 5-factor structure adequately fits these data and, of course, considerably better than the null model. In the hypothesized model, all factor loadings except two were over .45. The exceptions were values of 0.38 and 0.42. Also, t-values were significant ranging from 10.88 to 5.81 suggesting that the 39 items were appropriately grouped into the five hypothetical factors. Standardized factor loadings, means and standard deviations are presented in Table 3.

In order to examine the relationships among the 5 subscales, correlation coefficients were computed for all 10 pairs. The highest correlation was between Cues to Action and Benefits (.624). While this is a relatively high correlation for distinct subscales, 61% of the variance still remains unaccounted. This is consistent with the HBM conceptualization of Cues to Action as perceived immediate, short-term benefits. The correlation between Benefits and Susceptibility was -.529. All other correlations were below .50 (Table 4). Since the model does not hypothesize complete independence among factors, these findings seem to further support the utility of the HBMI with this population.

DISCUSSION

The high internal consistency for four of the five subscales supports the integrity of this instrument as a reasonable measure of the HBM constructs. The subscale with the lowest alpha coefficient, Cues to Action, may only occur as a distinct phenomenon when one actually decides to take action. This seems likely to occur within a rather restricted frame of reference which was not adequately isolated in this study. This restriction combined with the fact that this factor consisted of only three items may account for the low alpha value. Also, since all items among subscales seem to contribute to the total alpha coefficients, and they displayed relatively high factor loadings, it is reasonable to assume that items would remain fairly stable within these factors. These findings support the theoretical proposition that the individual items are most appropriately considered as sample measures of various HBM factors rather than isolated influences. This further supports the integrity of the HBMI. At the same time, it is unlikely that all possible items are included. This is particularly true when one considers the potential diversity of individuals making decisions about exercise. It is also unlikely that all items will be important for all groups. Nonetheless, the fact that they would remain relatively stable within factors supports the durability of the HBMI as a method of quantifying beliefs about Susceptibility, Benefits, Barriers, Social Influences and Cues to Action.

The intercorrelation between subscales was noted. The HBM does not, however, hypothesize uncorrelated factors. Several of the factors are quite logically related. For example, one who perceives high personal susceptibility is likely to be sensitized to the importance of benefits, and thus likely to respond more intensely to that factor as well. The subscale correlation of .529 reflects that relationship. A similar relationship can be argued for the clustering of Benefits, Social Influences, and Cues to Action. A global construct of benefits might accommodate all three factors. However, establishing separate factors allows one to more fully elaborate crucial components of the HBM. As noted above, these elements seemed stable enough to warrant consideration as distinct, though interrelated, factors.

The hypothesized factors were reflected by the model in spite of the homogeneity of age and other factors within the sample studied. While individual items may vary in their relevance to a given population, this analysis supports the utility of the HBM as a theoretical foundation for examining these decisions. These characteristics are particularly important when one considers the fact that the HBM is conceived in a way that lends itself to educational interventions. Thus, the HBM continues to be an attractive theoretical approach for understanding fitness decisions.

As Janz and Becker (1984) pointed out, research on the HBM has been plagued by weaknesses in instrumentation. The current study should be viewed as a preliminary test of the psychometric properties of an instrument reflecting the HBM constructs. While this study has begun to address that issue, future research is necessary in a variety of areas. Additional items need to be evaluated for inclusion in the various HBM factors. These items need to be tested on more heterogeneous samples. Also, other factors not currently accommodated by the model need to be identified and integrated. Finally, the effectiveness of educational interventions based on the Health Belief Model need to be evaluated in a more systematic, rigorous fashion.

REFERENCES

Becker, M., Maiman, L., Kirscht, J., Haefner, D., Drachman, R.L., & Taylor, D. (1979). In Hognes, R., Taylor, D., Snow, J. & Sackett, D. (Eds.), *Compliance in Health Care*. John Hopkins University Press, 78-109.

Becker, M. & Maimer, L. (1975). Sociobehavioral determinants of compliance with health and medical care recommendations. *Medical Care, 13,* 10-24.

Bentler, P.M. & Bonnet, D.G. (1980). Significance tests and goodness of fit in the analysis of co-variance structures. *Psychological Bulletin, 88,* 388-606.

Cronbach, L.J. (1951). Coefficient alpha and external structure of tests. *Psychometrika, 16,* 297-333.

deVries, H.A., Wiswell, R., Bulbulian, R. & Moritani, T. (1981). Tranquilizer effect of exercise. *American Journal of Physical Medicine, 60,* 57-66.

Griest, J.H., Klein, M., Eischens, R., Faris, J., Gruman, A. & Morgan, W.P. (1979). Running as treatment for depression. *Comprehensive Psychiatry, 20,* 41-54.

Iverson, D.C., Fielding, J., Grow, R. & Christenson, G. (1985). The promotion of physical activity in the United States population: The status of programs in medical worksite, community and school settings. *Public Health Reports, 100,* 212-224.

Janz, N.K. & Becker, N.H. (1984). The health belief model: A decade later. *Health Education Quarterly, 11,* 1-47.

Joreskog, K.G. (1969). A general approach to confirmatory maximum likelihood factor analysis. *Psychometrika, 34,* 1983-202.

Joreskog, K.G. & Sorbom, D. (1981). *LISREL-VI: Analysis of linear structural relationships by the method of maximum likelihood and least squares method.* Chicago International Education Services.

Joreskog, K.G. & Sorbom, D. (1984). *LISREL: Analysis of linear structural relationships by the method of maximum likelihood.* (Version VI). Mooresville, IN: Scientific Software.

Keeler, E.B., Manning, W.M., Newhouse, J., Sloss, E. & Wasserman, J. (1989). The external costs of a sedentary lifestyle. *Journal of the American Public Health Association, 79,* 975-982.

Morgan, W.P. (1979). Anxiety reduction following acute physical activity. *Psychiatric Annals, 9,* 141-147.

Morgan, W.P. (1981). Psychological benefits of physical activity. In Nagle, F.J. & Montogue, H.J. (Eds.), *Exercise, Health and Disease.* Springfield, Illinois: Charles C. Thomas, 299-314.

Rosenstock, I. (1974). Historical origins of the Health Belief Model. *Health Education Monographs, 2,* 328-335.

Slenker, S.E., Price, J.H., Roberts, S.M. & Jurs, S.G. (1984). Joggers versus nonexercisers: An analysis of knowledge, attitudes and beliefs about jogging. *Research Quarterly for Exercise and Sport, 55,* 371-378.

Steinhardt, M.A. & Corrier, K.M. (1989). Early and continued participation in a work-site health and fitness program. *Research Quarterly for Exercise and Sport, 60,* 117-126.

Stephens, T., Jacobs, Dr. R., & White, C.C. (1985). A descriptive epidemiology of leisure-time physical activity. *Public Health Reports, 100,* 147-158.

Taylor, C.B., Sallis, J.F. & Needle, R. (1985). The relation of physical activity and exercise to mental health. *Public Health Reports, 100,* 195-202.

Table 1

Internal Consistency Results

Subscale	# of Items	Alpha Coefficient	Item-Total r Range
Susceptibility	8	.86	.36–.75
Benefits	10	.89	.40–.75
Barriers	13	.85	.38–.65
Social Influences	5	.84	.53–.76
Cues to Action	3	.68	.39–.50

Table 2

Summary Statistics for Comfirmatory Factor Analysis

Index	5-Factor Value	Null Model Value
Coefficient of Determination	0.939	---
Chi-Square (df=692)	2103.51	6608.08
Ratio, Chi-Square: df	3.041	8.918
Goodness of Fit Index (GFI)	0.736	0.287
Adjusted GFI	0.702	0.250
Root Mean Square Residuals	0.170	0.497
Normed Fit Index ($\triangle$)	0.682	---

Table 3

Standardized Factor Loadings, Means, & Standard Deviations

Item	Loading	Mean	SD
Susceptibility			
overweight	.373	1.46	.98
nervousness or stress	.538	1.40	.82
coronary problems	.828	1.53	1.04
blood pressure	.758	1.47	.92
lack of energy	.699	1.88	1.29
colds or flu	.691	1.75	1.10
lung capacity	.542	1.35	.90
joint or muscle injureies	.797	3.19	1.66
Benefits of Exercise			
weight control	.477	6.24	1.20
provide frinedship	.857	5.23	1.69
relax or relieve tension	.938	6.18	1.18
sense of accomplishment	.790	6.39	.99
feel better	.767	6.46	.94
staying fit	.453	6.65	.63
more energy	.835	6.07	1.16
more patience/ understanding	1.035	4.86	1.67
more lung capacity	.663	6.38	.98
muscle tone	.419	6.57	.75
Barriers			
lack of time	.995	5.15	1.72
injuries	.927	4.84	1.73
work schedule	1.091	4.59	1.96
family responsibilities	.920	2.91	2.04
unsuitable weather	1.285	4.55	2.02
lack of desire	1.385	4.75	1.93
lack of energy	1.411	4.25	1.92
other preference	1.243	5.04	1.78
bad knees, back, etc.	.863	4.72	2.15
techniques confusing	.691	2.59	1.61
lack of self discipline	1.225	4.65	2.11
equipment choice confusing	.748	2.54	1.77
avoiding injuries confusing	.656	2.51	1.62
Social Influences			
spouse approved	.745	6.31	1.30
parents approved	1.003	6.26	1.30
friends approved	.959	6.30	1.09
physician approved	.721	6.18	1.29
co-workers approved	1.025	6.11	1.23
Cues to Action			
lose weight	1.067	5.95	1.63
get in shape	.772	6.43	1.03
experience stress	.951	5.47	1.71

Table 4

Subscale Correlations

	Susceptibility	Benefits	Barriers	Social Influences
Susceptibility	1.00			
Benefits	-0.529	1.00		
Barriers	0.261	-0.313	1.00	
Social Influences	-0.400	0.462	-0.173	1.00
Cues to Action	-0.264	0.624	-0.150	0.472

All correlations are significant at the $p < .001$ level

14

METHODOLOGICAL ISSUES IN EVALUATING THE IMPACT OF SCHOOL-BASED CLINICS

Michelle A. Bell
Mary Lou Balassone
Nancy Peterfreund

School-based clinics have become a popular approach to providing accessible, comprehensive health and mental health services to youth. Evaluating the impact of such clinics, however, presents many challenges. This paper, drawing from the experiences of the authors and other evaluators, suggests options for addressing the major methodological and practical considerations in planning and evaluation, developing the research design, implementing the study, and analyzing and reporting the findings. Specific topics include: assessing the purposes, audiences and resources for the evaluation; defining clinic objectives; specifying the program; defining the study population; choosing appropriate comparison groups; determining the timing and frequency of measurement; sources and methods of data collection; and special considerations in data analysis.

School-based clinics have become a popular approach to providing accessible, comprehensive health and mental health services to youth. Currently, there are more than 150 clinics in operation across the U.S. (Dryfoos, 1988). School-based clinics were developed both as a response to the health care needs of underserved adolescents and a recognition that the major health problems of adolescents - substance use, early pregnancy, sexually transmitted diseases, suicide and accidents - are not readily resolved within the standard medical care system (Millstein, 1988).

Services offered vary widely, but most often include primary care, physical exams, injury and trauma care, reproductive health services, mental health counseling, and health and nutritional education.

Evaluations of these programs are being conducted in order to assess two basic components of their effectiveness: (1) the impact of clinic services on student health-related behaviors and access to health care, and (2) the cost-effectiveness and viability of the clinics as a method of service delivery. While careful evaluation of clinic effectiveness is warranted, such research presents many methodological and practical challenges. Those challenges, and some possible solutions, are the focus of this discussion.

This paper examines issues related to the design and implementation of school-based clinic evaluations, with examples drawn from the published literature and from the authors' experience in evaluating the impact of a school-based health and mental health clinic in Washington state. It covers four major topics: planning the evaluation, developing an evaluation design, implementing the study, and analyzing and reporting the results.

A brief description of the longitudinal evaluation with which the authors were involved will provide a basis for discussion of these topics. The long-term purpose of the evaluation was to determine the impact of the clinic on students' physical and mental health status, health knowledge and behavior, and access to and utilization of needed health and mental health services. A major part of the evaluation design included collection of baseline and annual follow-up data in the school in which the clinic is located and in a comparable local school without a clinic. Self-administered, anonymous questionnaires were used to collect data from students in both schools. The questionnaires collected information in several areas: demographic characteristics; unmet health and mental health needs; knowledge related to contraception, sexually transmitted disease, and safety; drug and alcohol use; school success; and future goals. Follow-up surveys in the school with the clinic included questions on student satisfaction with clinic services, and reasons for use or non-use of the clinic. The evaluation also included bi-annual surveys of parents and teachers, annual reviews of records of student visits to the clinic, and review of attendance records from both schools. The process of planning and implementing this evaluation included consideration of a wide range of issues, many of which are described in the following discussion.

PLANNING THE EVALUATION: ASSESSING PURPOSES, AUDIENCES, AND RESOURCES

The initial step in an evaluation is an assessment of the purposes for which the research is being conducted, the audiences whose information needs must be met, and the resources available for carrying out the research activities. The results of this assessment provide the context for making decisions about the design of the study and the types of data to be collected.

Evaluations of school-based clinics, like many other program evaluations, must often address multiple purposes and audiences. Most evaluations have two basic purposes: to demonstrate the effectiveness of the program in achieving its objectives (outcome evaluation), and to provide information to help improve program administration and performance (process evaluation). Some have the additional purpose of comparing program costs and benefits. Information generated is often used as the basis for policy, funding, and program decisions.

Such evaluations address the information needs of a wide variety of audiences including funding bodies such as state and local governments or private foundations, clinic administrators and staff, school administrators, students who use the clinic and their parents, and the national audience of researchers and service providers.

Resources for conducting the evaluation also vary widely between projects. Some projects have substantial funding dedicated to a long-term evaluation effort while others have more modest resources, drawn primarily from the program budget and in-kind services.

Our evaluation had two primary audiences. City government, which provided the initial funding for the clinic, was interested in the cost of providing services and whether the clinic increased student access to health services. The city expected to use this information to determine whether to fund the clinic beyond the two-year demonstration period and to support additional clinics in schools throughout the city. The health department, which operates the clinic, wanted to determine the effectiveness of providing health services within the school setting, particularly for serving hard-to-reach adolescents.

There were, however, several other audiences with interest in the evaluation. The school district and the school which housed the clinic were interested in whether the clinic was helpful in reducing student absence due to illness or visits to health care providers, and in how well the clinic fit into the school setting without disrupting classroom activities. Clinic staff wanted ongoing information that would help them improve service delivery to students. Students, parents and the general community shared an interest in the evaluation since the results would help determine whether the clinic would continue to operate.

The multiple information needs generated by various purposes and audiences can be addressed by including several types and sources of data in the evaluation. In deciding what data should be included, evaluators must discuss with each audience its information needs and the form in which information is to be provided. Evaluators must also make clear to the audiences what research can reasonably be done with available resources. These discussions contribute to decisions regarding the evaluation design.

DEVELOPING THE EVALUATION DESIGN

The evaluation design provides the basis for determining whether a clinic has the intended impact upon a student population, which components of the clinic program were effective, which were not, and why. Three major tasks in developing the evaluation design include: defining the objectives for the clinic and selecting the variables or indicators by which the objectives will be measured; specifying the program components; and choosing a design to produce valid results, balancing methodological and practical considerations.

Defining Clinic Objectives: How is Success Measured?

Development of the evaluation design must begin with a clear definition of the objectives for the clinic and agreement on the criteria by which success will be determined. Various outcome measures have been adopted by researchers who have completed evaluations of school-based clinics.   Among the outcomes evaluated are: reduced rates of pregnancy among students (Edwards, Steinman, Arnold & Hakanson, 1980; Nowak, 1987; Zabin, Hirsch, Smith, Streett & Hardy, 1986); increased student utilization of health services (Welfare Research, 1987; Siegel & Kreible, 1987); decrease in substance use (Hill-Young, Kitzi, & Welch, 1987); decrease in school drop-outs (Nowak, 1987); improvement in mental health status (Hill-Young et al., 1987), and cost-effectiveness (Siegel & Kreible, 1987; Hill-Young et al., 1987). Process measures such as parent and student satisfaction with services (Siegel & Kreible, 1987) have also been used.

As these examples suggest, school-based clinics may have a variety of expected short- and long-term outcomes. Decisions about which outcomes to measure are mediated by consideration of time and resources available for the evaluation, and the impact a clinic can reasonably be expected to achieve during the study period. For example, one of the long-term objectives of our clinic was to improve student health status.   With only two years available for the study, we chose short-term indicators thought to lead to improved health status.   Short-term indicators included changes in student knowledge about such issues as prevention of pregnancy and sexually transmitted diseases, and changes in awareness of where to get care for health, mental health and drug problems. Intermediate-term indicators included changes in access to and utilization of health care for specific problems.

At the time the evaluation is designed there may be difficulty in specifying all of the clinic's expected outcomes due to uncertainty about services to be offered in the future, availability of funds, staffing patterns, or the focus of future health education campaigns. A good rule of thumb is to measure as many effects as are relevant to clinic goals and services to ensure that all outcomes of interest are included in the evaluation. Variables for which there has been no intervention can be eliminated at later data collection points.

Specifying the Program: What is the Intervention?

The next task is to specify the nature of the program activities by which the objectives will be achieved. Program specification assures that the outcomes selected for the evaluation are indeed related to program activities.

Program specification also enables the evaluator to identify variables for the process evaluation. By clearly identifying, measuring and monitoring process variables the evaluator will be better able to explain which attributes of the program led to the observed effects.

Once program activities and expected outcomes have been specified, a model describing how the program is intended to work can be outlined. Such a model permits examination of the relationship between process and outcome variables, makes explicit the assumptions that underlie the program, and permits the evaluator to test the validity of those assumptions (Weiss, 1972).

Table 1 illustrates the use of a program model with a format adapted from Jones, Namerow, and Philliber (1986) and variables from our evaluation. The table displays the program inputs (staff, facilities and funding) that produce program outputs (health and mental health services) and lead to the expected outcomes. We used the model to test the assumptions of the program. For example, one assumption was that staffing the clinic with a counselor (program input) to provide mental health and drug/alcohol counseling (program output) would result in increased student awareness of where to get counseling (short-term outcome), use of that service (intermediate outcome), and improved mental health status (long-term outcome). The evaluation design included measures of these process and outcome variables.

CHOOSING THE RESEARCH DESIGN: MAJOR CONSIDERATIONS

It is beyond the scope of this paper to outline every possible evaluation design; that information is readily available in textbooks devoted to the topic (Campbell & Stanley, 1963; Rossi & Freeman, 1985). Instead, the discussion highlights the major considerations and trade-offs that face evaluators in defining the study population, selecting appropriate comparison groups, and setting the timing and frequency of measurement.

In addressing each of these design tasks, the evaluator must give special consideration to issues of internal and external validity. External validity is the extent to which the findings can be generalized to other settings and reproduced in similar settings. External validity can be limited by the social and demographic characteristics of the study population, lack of program specificity, and interaction between the intervention and self-selection of students who use it. External validity is best addressed by clearly specifying the population, program, and study methods and limitations.

Internal validity is the extent to which research results can be attributed to the presence of a school-based clinic rather than to extraneous factors. Four types of extraneous factors are particularly important to evaluations of school-based clinics: community and school events that are unrelated to the clinic but influence student outcome measures; maturation of students that produces behavioral changes closely related to clinic activities; characteristics of students which predispose them to either use or not use the clinic; and movement of students into and out of the school due to promotions, transfers, and drop-outs that change the composition of the student body on whom clinic outcomes are measured. Threats to internal validity must be addressed in each aspect of the research design.

Defining the Study Population

Defining the study population involves several decisions: whether to study the entire student body of a school in which a clinic is located or just those who use the clinic; how to define and measure relevant population sub-groups; and how to track changes in the student body due to absences, drop-outs, and transfers.

Evaluating the effectiveness of a clinic on the total student body of a school is thought by some researchers to provide the most rigorous test of the program by measuring the effects on all students who are eligible to participate (Zabin & Hirsch, 1988). Measuring all students in the school also affords the opportunity to compare the characteristics of clinic users and non-users, and to collect other information useful for a process evaluation.

Other researchers suggest that a more reasonable test is to measure a clinic's effectiveness only among those students who choose to avail themselves of its services (Kirby, Waszak & Ziegler, 1989). Experience indicates that only about half of the students in a school actually use clinic services. Effects may be underestimated if clinic impact is measured against the total student body due to inadequate statistical power. However, focusing the evaluation only on clinic users introduces selection bias since clinic users are a self-selected group.

The optimal approach to defining the sample is best determined by the purposes of the evaluation and the importance of demonstrating statistically significant changes. In our study, for example, we were interested in evaluating changes in health care access and utilization among all students in the school as well as assessing the characteristics of clinic users and non-users, so we collected data on the total student population. While we applied statistical tests in the analysis, we were also concerned with examining the direction, magnitude and consistency of changes as well as with statistical significance.

Once the study population has been defined, the evaluator must define relevant population sub-groups. Most of these sub-group definitions will derive from the specific objectives of the clinic. For example, our program school has several ethnic groups within the student body for whom we wished to assess clinic impact, so ethnicity was measured in student data collected.

Evaluations that assess clinic effects over two or more years should include a measure of student exposure to the program. Students experience different exposure to the clinic as a result of their movement into and out of the school. For example, ninth graders and transfer students who enter a school during the second year of the clinic program have less exposure than students who were present during both the first and second years. Measuring exposure enables the evaluator to determine whether the impact of clinic services is incremental. We adopted a simple measure of exposure by asking students their present grade and the year they entered the program school. Grade alone is not sufficient to measure exposure since students transfer into a school at various times during the clinic program.

The evaluator must also determine a method for tracking changes in the study population over time. Changes occur as a result of the normal progression of students into and through the school, and as a result of absences, drop-outs, and transfers. Significant changes in the study population between the time of baseline and follow-up measures can compromise study results. Student enrollment and attendance data can be used to track these changes, but evaluators must determine how these records are kept in the schools studied.

Selecting Appropriate Comparison Groups

The next task is to select one or more groups against which evaluation results can be compared. Use of appropriate comparison groups enables the evaluator to distinguish the effects of the clinic from community events or maturation of students. Various types of comparison groups are discussed briefly and illustrated with examples from completed evaluations.

Designs using one or more comparison schools without clinic programs have been used in some outcome evaluations (Kirby et al., 1989; Zabin & Hirsch, 1986). The objective in selecting a comparison school is to find one that is as similar as possible to the program school. Sociodemographic characteristics of the students such as socioeconomic status and race/ethnicity are always considered, since family income and cultural values are likely to affect students' use of health care. The proportion of students receiving free or reduced cost lunches can be used as a proxy for socioeconomic status. School attendance information, such as rate of absences and drop-outs; and school performance data, such as standardized test scores, can also be used in selecting comparison schools.

Practical considerations in choosing a comparison school include finding out whether changes are anticipated in that school's program that might affect the variables of interest. A school that plans to expand nursing services, for example, would not be a good candidate since students' use of health services could be affected by increased availability.

Regardless of the care taken in selecting a comparison school, a perfect match will not be achieved. Statistical controls, which attain comparability of the two groups by holding constant the differences between them, can be applied at the time of data analysis for those characteristics that are explicitly measured. However, there will remain unmeasured differences between the schools that could affect the evaluation results.

Evaluators have used other comparison groups to assess impact on specific variables. Edwards et al., (1980), in examining the impact of a school-based clinic on student pregnancy, compared students in the program school with teenagers using other family planning clinics on variables such as continuation of contraceptive use, repeat pregnancy, and school continuation. Siegel and Kreible (1987), in determining the cost effectiveness of school-based clinics, compared the cost of physical exams given in the school clinic with the cost of exams by private providers in the community. Nowak (1987), in investigating the impact of a clinic on school performance, compared standardized test scores of students in the program school with those in other schools in the district. Evaluation results can be strengthened through use of carefully selected comparison groups.

Frequency and Timing of Measurement

Decisions regarding the frequency and timing of data collection are governed by both substantive and practical considerations. Data must be collected frequently enough to capture changes in age-related behaviors such as sexual activity and drug use, but not so frequently as to introduce testing effects.

Testing effects can occur when students are given the same data-collection instrument at close intervals; differences observed between the two tests may occur as a result of the test itself rather than the clinic. Practical considerations, such as the resources available for the evaluation, also affect the frequency of measurement. The evaluator must balance all of these considerations in deciding on the frequency of measurement.

We chose to collect data annually. Annual surveys provide reasonable assurance of capturing age-related behaviors. However, they require more resources than less frequent data collection, and may not show large changes on the variables of interest between measurement points. Students may become bored with repeated surveys and their responses may be affected. At least one evaluation has collected data biannually (Kirby et al., 1989). That study found significant changes in the characteristics of the student body as a result of general changes in the community between the two measurement points. The experience of Kirby et al. suggests that annual measurement may be preferable in schools or communities undergoing rapid changes in population characteristics such as income which could confound evaluation results.

Timing of data collection must also be considered. School populations change over the academic year. Enrollment is largest early in the school year and falls off dramatically by the end of the year as a result of transfers and drop-outs. Drop-outs may have higher rates of pregnancy, school failure, drug use and other problems that are the focus of clinic activities. Collection of baseline data in the fall and follow-up data in the spring could result in "improvement" on these variables that was attributable to drop-outs rather than to the clinic. For this reason, data should be collected at the same time each year to ensure that similar students are included in the sample. Late autumn has been suggested as a reasonable time, since enrollment is stable at that time (Zabin & Hirsch, 1988).

As the foregoing discussion suggests, developing the evaluation design involves a series of methodological and practical trade-offs that the evaluator must weight carefully before implementing the study.

IMPLEMENTING THE EVALUATION

Sources of Data and Methods of Collection

Evaluations of school-based clinics can use data from multiple sources: students, clinic records, school staff, parents, school records, and community-based statistics. Use of multiple data sources permits measurement of both process and outcome variables as well as comparison of findings derived from different sources. This section discusses the types of process and outcome data that can be collected from these various sources. Methodological problems and tactics that can be used to resolve them are highlighted.

Self-administered surveys of students are commonly used to measure clinic impact (Kirby et al., 1989; Zabin & Hirsch, 1988). Surveys typically contain questions on demographic characteristics; health and mental health problems; utilization of health services; attitudes, knowledge and behavior related to health issues such as substance abuse, pregnancy, sexually transmitted disease, vehicle safety, and violence; and school success and future goals.

For our evaluation, we administered an anonymous baseline survey to all students in the program and comparison schools in the fall before the clinic opened. We administered follow-up surveys to all students in both schools near the end of the school year and again at the end of the second year of the clinic program. Clinic impact was measured by assessing changes on the outcome variables for students in the program and comparison schools.

Information on process measures can also be collected using surveys administered in the program school after the clinic is introduced. Surveys can include items to measure use or non-use of the clinic, reasons for which students used the clinic or chose not to use it, and satisfaction with clinic staff and the services provided. In our follow-up survey, we asked students in the program school how the clinic could be improved, and whether there were any services they would like to have added. The responses provided information that was helpful in refining the clinic's services. Such information can also provide insight on the characteristics of users and non-users that can be helpful in marketing clinic services.

Some caveats are needed regarding the use of self-administered questionnaires. Self reported data may contain biases that result from the student's deliberate distortion of responses, failure to comprehend the questions, or inaccurate recall of the events asked about. Distortion of responses by adolescents due to overreporting or underreporting of behaviors such as drug use has been demonstrated in about 10% of subjects (Winters, Stinchfield, Henly & Schwartz, in press). Some distortion bias can be controlled by using data cleaning procedures such as those discussed below. In addition, data derived from other sources may also be used to corroborate survey data.

Subject comprehension of questions and recall of events can be improved by careful instrument design. Student reading ability and language skills must be taken into account in the design of self-administered questionnaires. Both our program and comparison schools include students for whom English is a second language as well as other students with limited reading skills. Therefore, the survey instrument had to be constructed to accommodate the skill levels of these students. Language in the questionnaire was kept as simple as possible, alternative terms were given for things some students might not be familiar with (e.g., urination, peeing), and the total length of the survey was limited to permit completion by slower readers. Questions were ordered so that those most important to the evaluation were placed near the beginning in order to increase the opportunity for slower readers to complete those items. The questionnaire was pre-tested with heterogeneous groups of students. Survey staff discussed the questionnaire with the students, item by item, to clarify the wording and find terms that were understandable to everyone. When the survey was administered, teachers in classrooms with large numbers of students with low reading skills read the questionnaire aloud while students completed it. All of these steps were taken to assure that the survey results would be valid and representative of all students in the program and comparison schools.

Clinic Records

Clinic records provide useful information for the process evaluation. Characteristics of students who use clinic services; the types of health problems seen and treated by staff; the number and frequency of medical, counseling or other visits to the clinic; and information on referrals and follow-up can be derived from clinic records. Aggregate clinic data can also be used to validate the results of student surveys; if non-anonymous surveys are used, survey and clinic data can be linked for specific individuals. Clinic data can also provide essential information for cost analyses.

The major limitation of clinic records as a source of evaluation data is that they are available only for direct users of clinic services, and cannot be used to measure effects of the clinic on knowledge or health behavior among all students. Clinic records are best used, therefore, in conjunction with other measures.

If clinic records are to be used in the evaluation, the system for collecting and analyzing data must be designed for this purpose and staff must be trained to complete the data collection form accurately and consistently. Our clinic is operated by the county health department which uses a computerized data system to maintain records. It was necessary to modify the system to accommodate codes for clinic services, and to train clinic staff in use of the system.

School Staff Surveys

School staff surveys can be used to monitor the functioning of the clinic within the school setting. Such process evaluation information is important because program success often depends on continuing support from teachers and administrators. Our evaluation included a self-administered survey, given to all school staff at the end of the school year, which asked about referrals made to the clinic, impact of the clinic on classroom attendance and activities, teacher satisfaction with services to students, and how the clinic's services might be improved. The survey was anonymous and invited comments through several open-ended questions. The results provided insights on the way teachers and staff viewed the clinic, suggestions for improving both the process and content of clinic services, and creative suggestions for integrating clinic staff into classroom activities.

Parent surveys are also an important source of process evaluation data. These surveys can measure parent support and attitudes which are critical to the success of the clinic. Parents are instrumental in defining the clinic's program of services, and must give written permission for their teenagers to use the clinic. Once the clinic is in operation, feedback from parents regarding the role of the clinic in meeting their teenagers' health care needs can guide further development of services. Our evaluation included a mailed, self-administered survey to parents of clinic users which was conducted at the end of the first year of clinic operation. The survey asked parents' opinions on the quality of clinic staff and services, the services considered to be essential, and any additional services that the clinic should offer. Demographic information enabled the evaluators to interpret parents' responses.

Clinic staff are also an important source of process evaluation information. Providing health services within a school setting is likely to be a new experience for most health providers, who must simultaneously address the health problems specific to their adolescent clients and the interprofessional and organizational issues inherent in the setting. Clinic staff can provide information on such issues as clinic flow, factors that facilitate or inhibit service provision, and the need for changes in the mix of services offered. Data can be collected from clinic staff using interviews or written surveys.

School attendance records can provide useful information on the populations of both program and comparison schools regarding absentee, drop-out, and suspension rates. Attendance information has at least two applications to the evaluation of school-based clinics. First, school attendance is directly related to the goals of most clinic programs: to improve the health of students so they are able to remain in school, and to provide services on-site so students do not have to miss school to get health care. Attendance data can be used to evaluate success in achieving these goals, provided that reasons for absence can be ascertained and only changes in health-related absences are used to evaluate the clinic program. A second use for school attendance data is to estimate bias in survey results due to absentees. Such data may be limited, however, by inconsistent reporting procedures and failure to track absentees and drop outs. Evaluators should check with schools to determine how information is compiled prior to its use.

Community indicators can be used to evaluate clinic programs that have such goals as reducing teen pregnancy or crime rates in the school's catchment area. Several factors limit the use of community indicators. First, calculating rates requires careful determination of the appropriate denominator, that is, the community or population of interest. Second, current data for either the numerator or denominator may not be available or may not be comparable for the areas in which the program and comparison schools are located. Third, community indicators such as pregnancy rates are not sensitive to the small changes a school-based clinic is likely to affect. For these reasons, community indicators are best used to supplement other sources of evaluation data.

Record of events in the community and schools that could influence evaluation results should be kept by evaluators. Such events might include media campaigns targeting specific health issues or accidents that receive media coverage. For example, three students from our program school were killed in a car crash three months before the clinic opened. This event was reflected in an unusually high percentage of students who reported loss of a close friend or family member in the past year. Evaluators' knowledge of the event prevented misinterpretation of data.

Practical Considerations

Evaluations of school-based clinics must consider issues that derive from the educational setting and the social-political environment in which schools operate. The first issue concerns the need to enlist and maintain the cooperation of administrators, teachers, and students in the program and comparison schools. Surveys of students take up class time. To minimize disruption - and maximize the quality of data collected - evaluators must prepare carefully for survey administration. They may also wish to consider offering incentives to compensate for the time and effort involved in data collection, particularly in the comparison school where no clinic services are offered.

Second, parental consent may be required for students to participate in data-collection activities. Most school districts use passive consent procedures in which parents are notified of the survey and given the option of withdrawing their child from participation. Some districts, however, require active consent when surveys contain sensitive questions regarding students' personal behavior such as sexual or illegal activities. In those districts signed permission slips must be obtained from parents before students can participate in a survey. Survey results may be biased if a substantial proportion of students fail to return the slips and cannot participate.

Finally, school districts may make substantial changes in policies and procedures over time which will affect the evaluation effort. For example, Kirby et al., (1989) report that one school district changed its policies on parental consent from passive to active procedures between data-collection periods. School districts may also change procedures for assigning students to schools, thus affecting the student populations of program and comparison schools. Evaluators must be prepared to make adjustments in sampling and data collection plans as a result of such changes.

DATA ANALYSIS AND REPORTING

Data Coding and Cleaning

Evaluations using self-administered questionnaires for data collection must include data coding and cleaning procedures to assure internal consistency and reliability. Our study employed several steps in the data cleaning process. First, coders who prepared the data for computer entry looked for obviously strange responses and made note of them. For example, surveys were noted on which every item in a list of serious life events was checked, or responses appeared to be checked randomly. Evaluation staff then looked at the original data and decided whether to eliminate the entire questionnaire or to exclude problematic responses from further analysis. In a very few instances, inconsistencies resulted from simple mistakes and were resolved by making minor adjustments in the data. This procedure was guided by the consistent application of decision rules.

The next step, carried out when all of the data had been entered into the computer and initial frequencies had been run, was to institute a series of inter-item consistency checks. Questionnaires with inconsistent responses were identified, examined, and either retained or eliminated from further analysis. Data cleaning must be repeated on each set of survey data collected, although computer programs for consistency checks, once written, can be used with new data.

Data Analysis

Data analysis is guided by the process and outcome measures adopted for the evaluation. Analysis also involves bringing together data collected from various sources. This section illustrates the approach taken in our evaluation.

Outcomes - the impact of the clinic on student knowledge, awareness, clinic use, and health/mental health status - were determined from analysis of the student surveys. We compared student responses on the baseline and follow-up surveys for the program and comparison schools, and measured the magnitude of change for each of the outcome variables. Statistical tests were used to determine whether the changes were significant.

Statistical techniques were used to control for differences between the program and comparison schools. Although the specific control variables must be determined for each evaluation, the variables of gender, ethnicity, age, and income are usually considered.

Sub-group analyses using data from follow-up surveys of the program school can provide insights on the types of students who use (and do not use) the clinic. For example, we assessed differences between clinic users and non-users with respect to demographic characteristics, sources of health care and problems encountered in getting health care. This analysis indicated that students who used the clinic were those most in need of health care (Balassone, Bell & Peterfreund, 1990). Other special analyses might focus on student alcohol and drug use, mental health status, or nutritional habits, depending on the data collected. These analyses contribute to the process analysis, and are useful in refining and marketing clinic services.

Process data from surveys of students, teachers and parents were analyzed to determine knowledge of and satisfaction with the clinic. Clinic records were compiled to show patterns and frequency of use, types of diagnoses, treatment and referrals, and characteristics of students using the clinic.

The final step in the analysis is to integrate and compare data from multiple sources. Clinic records can be compared with items from student surveys which ask about health problems, types of care received, and reasons for using the clinic. Teacher and parent survey data can be compared with student data to identify common issues and concerns related to clinic services. Data from various sources should present a consistent and coherent picture of clinic impact (Kirby, 1989).

Reporting the Results

The presence of multiple audiences for evaluations of school-based clinics often requires preparation of multiple reports, each designed to answer the questions of a specific group. We prepared comprehensive reports for the mayor and city council, internal reports for the health department, focused reports for clinic staff, summaries for the students and teachers of the program school and the general community, and presentations and research papers for local and national audiences of health professionals. Each report or presentation focused on the interests of the particular audience.

Local news media can serve as another forum for presenting evaluation results. We held a press conference that featured the mayor and representatives of the school district and health department to announce results from the first year of clinic operation and support for continuation. Media events must be carefully orchestrated, however, to assure that information about clinic services and outcomes are reported accurately and completely.

Graphics and charts can be effective means for presenting data and can be used with many different types of audiences. Selected comments from the student, teacher, and parent surveys can be used to illustrate attitudes toward the clinic and ideas for improving services, and add a personal dimension to the data.

CONCLUSION

While the evaluation of school-based clinics presents many challenges to the researcher, carefully designed and executed studies are needed to answer basic questions about the impact and cost-effectiveness of clinic programs in addressing adolescent health concerns.   We have presented some of the major considerations in planning and carrying out such evaluations in the hope that our experience, and that of others, will contribute to future evaluation efforts.

REFERENCES

Balassone, M.L., Bell, M.A., & Peterfreund, N. Evaluation of a school-based health and mental health clinic: Comparison of users and non-users. *Journal of Adolescent Health Care,* in press.

Brindis, C., Korenbrot, C., Selzer, L., & Erickson, P. Fostering and evaluating school-based comprehensive health services for secondary schools in California: Preliminary results of needs assessments. Paper presented to the American Public Health Association, October 1987.

Campbell, D.T. & Stanley, J.C. (1963). *Experimental and quasi-experimental designs for research.* Boston, Massachusetts: Houghton Mifflin.

Dryfoos, J.G. (1988). School-based clinics: Three years of experience. *Family Planning Perspectives, 20,* 193-200.

Edwards, L., Steinman, M., Arnold, K. & Hakanson, E. (1980). Adolescent pregnancy prevention services in high school clinics. *Family Planning Perspectives, 12,* 6-15.

Futterman, R. & Lopez, M. (1987). Evaluating a comprehensive school-based clinic program: Baseline findings. New York: Columbia University, Center for Population and Family Health.

Hill-Young, J., Kitzi, G. & Welch, Q.B. (1987). The school-based clinic as a health promotion tool to improving the health status of inner city black youth. Presented to the Black Caucus of Health Workers.

Jones, J.E., Namerow, P.B. & Philliber, S.G. (1986). Strategies for evaluating a contraceptive service for teenagers. *HCMR, 11,* 41-46.

Kirby, D., Waszak, C.S. & Ziegler, J. (1989). An Assessment of Six School-Based Clinics: Services, Impact and Potential. Washington, D.C.: Center for Population Options, Support Center for School-Based Clinics.

Millstein, S.G. (1988). The potential of school-linked centers to promote adolescent health and development. Washington, D.C.: Carnegie Council on Adolescent Development.

Nowak, N. (1987). Shanks health center evaluation, final report: First year of program operation. Tallahassee: Florida State University, Center for Human Services Policy and Administration.

Riggs, S. & Cheng, T. (1988). Adolescents' willingness to use a school-based clinic in view of expressed health concerns. *Journal of Adolescent Health Care, 9,* 208-213.

Rossi, P.H. & Freeman, H.E. (1985). Evaluation: A Systematic Approach. Beverly Hills: Sage Publications.

Siegel, L. & Kreible, T. (1987). Evaluation of school-based high school health services. *Journal of School Health, 57*, 323-325.

Weiss, C. (1972). *Evaluation research: Methods of assessing program effectiveness.* Englewood Cliffs: Prentice-Hall.

Welfare Research, Inc. (1987). Health services for high school students: Short-term assessment of the New York City high school-based clinics. New York: Welfare Research, Inc.

Winters, K.C., Stinchfield, R.D., Henly, G.A. & Schwartz, R.H. Accuracy of adolescent self-report of alcohol and drug involvement. *The International Journal of Addictions*, in press.

Zabin, L.S. & Hirsch, M.B. (1988). *Evaluation of pregnancy prevention programs in the school context.* Lexington, Massachusetts: Lexington Books.

Zabin, L.S., Hirsch, M.B., Smith, E.A., Strett, R. & Hardy, J.B. (1986). Evaluation of a pregnancy prevention program for urban teenagers. *Family Planning Perspectives, 18*, 119-126.

Program Model of a School-Based Clinic

INPUTS	OUTPUTS	OUTCOMES
Staff	**Health**	**Short-term**
Physician	Exam	Knowledge
Nurse practitioner	Diagnosis	Awareness
Counselor	Treatment	
Receptionist/Health	Laboratory	**Intermediate**
Aide	Referral	Clinic use
	Health education	Satisfaction
Facilities		
	Mental Health	**Long-Term**
Funding	Assessment	Improved
	Counseling	health/mental
	Referral	health status

Adapted from J.G. Jones, P.B. Namerow, and S.G. Philliber. Strategies for Evaluating a Contraceptive Service for Teenagers. HCMR, 1986, 11, 41-46.

15

CONSTRUCT VALIDITY AND RE-ASSESSMENT OF THE RELIABILITY OF THE HEALTH CONCERN QUESTIONNAIRE

Ruth C. Engs

The Health Concern Questionnaire was developed almost 20 years ago (Engs, 1970) and has been used by both personal health classroom instructors and researchers. In this time some of the terminology for certain items have changed. A more serious limitation of its usefulness was that construct validity was not initially determined, resulting in the inability to calculate a total mean health concern score. Thus the purpose of the study was to update the terminology, determine construct validity, and revalidate the internal consistency of the instrument.

The first step in this procedure was to have a panel of individuals who had taught personal health classes suggest changes in terminology. The next step was to accomplish a factor analysis to determine underlying themes using an eigenvalue of 1, resulting in nine factors. Factor 1 contained 27 of the items and accounted for 31% of the variance. Since there was no underlying theme of health areas for any of the factors, a two-factor solution with an eigenvalue of 2 was used. The results indicated factor 1 contained 33% of the variance and included 31 items dealing with issues of personal, social, and mental health problems. The remaining items in factor 2 contributed 7% of the variance containing sexuality and personal health items. Further analysis indicated a correlation between the two primary factors was positive (r=.6). This relationship enabled the collapse of the 50 items into one factor and the feasibility of computing total mean health concern score.

Cronbach's alpha (r=.96), Spearman-Brown's split half technique (r=.92) and Guttman's split half technique (r=.92) all revealed high reliability coefficients. The item reliability of each of the 50 items correlated with the total mean score and revealed positive coefficients. They ranged from r=.43 to r=.73.

303

In summary, current terminology for the Health Concern Questionnaire has been added. A total mean health concern score can be ascertained and the instrument shows high internal consistency homogeneity.

The *Health Concern Questionnaire (HCQ)* has been used over the past 20 years by educators to rank college students' concerns about health-related issues. This information is then used for curriculum planning in personal health classes. It has also been used in research studies attempting to determine current health concerns (Schaaldt and Engs, 1971), health concerns in relationship to specific health areas (Engs, 1983), changes in health concerns over time (Goodrow, 1977; Engs, 1985), and cross-cultural aspects of health concerns (Engs and Badr, 1984). It has also been used in unpublished studies by graduate students. However, the HCQ is now about 20 years old. It was originally developed as a masters thesis between 1968 and 1970 (Engs, 1970). Since it is still used by health educators both in the classroom and for research purposes, it needs to be updated. Items in the original questionnaire involved physical, mental, and social concerns at the personal and societal level. Topics on the HCQ included human sexuality, alcohol and other drugs, accidents, environmental issues, social conflict, mental health, personal health, sexually transmitted disease, and chronic illnesses.

A limitation of the questionnaire was that it could only rank students' concerns about various health topics, rather than providing a total health concern score. A total score would make the HCQ more useful. This limitation exists because factor analysis, which would determine underlying themes for the possible calculation of a single score, had not been conducted during initial scale development. Moreover, a basic assumption, according to Durkheims' (1951) theory of social change, suggests that as society changes people's attitudes and beliefs also change. This could lead to changes in terminology and concerns about a variety of health matters. For more accuracy in gauging students' concerns about health items, current terms were needed.

Therefore, the purpose of this study was to revise the original instrument in terms of current terminology and concerns. Additionally, construct validity of the scale items would be assessed to determine the feasibility of being able to sum the items in a manner which would result in a total health concern score. Finally, the health concerns of students in the latter part of the 1980s would be ranked; this information may serve as a guideline for curriculum planning.

METHODS

Sample

All students enrolled in the small section (<50 students) personal health classes at a large midwestern university during the 1988 academic year were asked to volunteer to participate in the study. This course enrolls students from all undergraduate majors and is considered a life science elective. Procedures for administering the questionnaire conformed to the Human Subjects Review committee protocol. Approximately 30 questionnaires were unusable due to improper completion. The resulting convenience sample contained 388 undergraduate students (92% response rate). Power analysis indicated this sample size had enough power to detect significant differences (Cohen, 1988).

Degree of Concern

Students indicated their degree of concern for each item by using the number "5" for Extremely Concerned, "4" for Very Concerned, "3" for Moderately Concerned, "2" for Mildly Concerned, and "1" for Not Concerned. To interpret the results for comparisons across these groups, each item was given a value range. "Extremely Concerned" = 5.00-4.56, "Very Concerned" = 4.5-3.56, etc.

Various procedures (discussed below) were utilized to assess content validity, construct validity, item reliability, and internal consistency.

Content Validity

The instrument was first tested for content or face validity to determine if it still measured what it was intended to test. To carry out this procedure it was initially reviewed by four doctoral students and three faculty members who had taught personal health courses. They were asked to update terms, to clarify confusing items, and to comment on the apparent validity of each item.

After examination by these individuals, several items were changed. "Venereal Disease" was changed to "Sexually Transmitted Diseases other than AIDS." "Vietnam War" as a current crisis issue was replaced by "AIDS," "Atomic Warfare" was updated to "Nuclear Warfare," and "Vietnam Combat" was changed to "Combat."

The resulting form was administered to 97 personal health students during the 1987 spring term. They were asked to comment and to clarify items which were not easily understood. No items were changed.

Construct Validity

A search for underlying themes was conducted using the factor analysis technique. A minimum eigenvalue of 1.0 and the orthogonal rotation solution (varimax) procedure using the SPSSX package was used (Norusis, 1987). This procedure was also carried out to determine if a simple method for summing all of the items resulting in a total health concern score would be possible.

Items Reliability

Item reliability of each item in relationship to the total score would be carried out using the Pearson Correlation analysis depending upon the results of the factor analysis. This procedure would be accomplished if the factor analysis indicated that either a simple regression equation for determining a total score could be utilized or if the individual items could be summed for a total health concern score.

Internal Consistency and Homogeneity

To examine the internal consistency reliability of the 50 item questionnaire, the Spearman-Brown prophecy formula for equal lengths test was accomplished. Cronbach's alpha measurement of homogeneity was calculated. The Guttman's split-half technique for reliability of the instrument was also calculated. All these procedures were accomplished using the SPSSX program (Norusis, 1987).

Ranking of Health Concerns

To rank the items, the highest to lowest mean score of each item was determined. In case of ties the item with the greatest variance was ranked first.

RESULTS

Construct Validity

Factor analysis using principle component analysis with an orthogonal (varimax) rotation solution and a minimum eigenvalue of 1 as the cut-off point for the totaled factors, indicated the instrument contained nine factors. Factor 1 explained 33.3% of the variance. It contained 27 of the 50 items. Factor 1 contained miscellaneous items ranging from "liver diseases" to "masturbation" and involved personal, social, physical, and mental health items. Factor 2 contained 19 items with five of the items relating to sexual matters while the other items identified other personal health problems. This factor accounted for 7% of the variance. Factor 3 contained three items related to war or pollution. The other factors contained one item each. It was decided to keep the three items from factor 3 in this scale as they are important current environmental health problems. However, it could be easily argued that these items should be deleted and only the 46 items in factor 1 and factor 2 be retained. Because no clear underlying themes were found and because of the numerous resulting factors, the analysis was recalculated with a forced two factor solution. This was accomplished by using a minimum eigenvalue of 2.

This resulted in Factor 1 containing 31 items (explaining 33.3% of the variance) and factor 2 containing the remaining items (explaining 7% of the variance) (Table 1). The correlation between the two factors was positive (r=.58).

Because of the high association between the two factors and because both factors appeared to be a mix of personal, mental, social, and environmental issues, it was concluded that the test of 50 items could be collapsed into one factor. This results in the ability to sum all of the 50 items for a total health concern score.

Homogeneity and Internal Consistency

The Cronbach alpha test for homogeneity of the 50 item instrument revealed an extremely high alpha coefficient (r=.96). The Guttman's split half technique procedure resulted in a high reliability coefficient (r=.92). Likewise the Spearman-Brown held technique for equal length tests revealed a highly significant (p<.001) reliability coefficient (r=.92). These high reliability coefficients infer that the test halves are highly correlated and the questionnaire has high internal consistency.

The mean score for the questionnaire was 118 (SD=32). The 93 individuals one standard deviation above the mean (>150) were considered to have a high degree of concern about these items, while the 114 individuals one standard deviation below the mean (<86) were believed to have a low degree of concern. The total health concern score can range from 50 to 200.

Item Analysis

Item analysis for each of the 50 questions with the total health concern mean score revealed that all items had a reliability coefficient above r=.43. The reliability coefficients ranged from r=.43 to r=.72.

Ranking of Concerns

The highest ranking health concern was AIDS with a mean score of 3.5 that fell in the range of "moderate" concern. Since this is a fatal disease with no cure, it was encouraging to find that students do in fact feel concerned about this condition. Of course, it is unknown if students in this sample who are concerned then engage in positive prevention methods. The other top ten items included a mixture of social, mental, and personal concerns. They consisted of: the future (death, what I'll be like in 10 or 15 years), sexuality (birth control, use of contraceptives, sexually transmitted diseases other than AIDS), chronic disease (cancer), accidents (auto accidents), overweight, and nuclear warfare. For these top ten concerns students in this sample indicated only "moderate" concern for any item with the mean scores ranging from 3.5 to 2.9 (Table 2).

Two of the leading causes of death among youth, namely auto accidents and cancer, were included among the top ten concerns. On the other hand, suicide, another leading cause of death, ranked 26th. Perhaps this problem is not being thoroughly discussed in mental health units of personal health courses, and students may not be aware that suicide is a problem among youth.

SUMMARY AND CONCLUSION

The determination of construct validity of the Health Concern Questionnaire has resulted in a more usable instrument for a variety of situations. Determining a high correlation between the two major factors underlying the instrument enables the researcher or educator to administer the questionnaire and obtain a total health concern score. Re-assessment of the internal consistency of the instrument demonstrated the questionnaire is highly reliable. Moreover, the researcher or educator can determine the degree of concern for each individual item by assessing its mean score and then ascertain the ranking of all health items. For this sample of students, AIDS was the item of most concern. Among the top ten areas were issues of sexuality, leading causes of death among this age group, and potential future health issues.

Acknowledgement

This project was funded by Indiana University. I would like to thank David Koceja for assistance with the statistical procedures and programming.

REFERENCES

Cohen, J. (1988). *Statistical power analysis for the behavioral sciences (second edition).* Hillsdale, N.J.: Lawrence Erlbaum Associates.

Durkheim, E. (1951). *Le Suicide.* Trans. by Spaulding, J. and Simpson, G. New York: Free Press.

Engs, R.C. (1985, June/July). Health concerns over time: The apparent stability. *Health Education, 3-6.*

Engs, R.C. & Badr, L.H. (1983). The health concerns of young American and Egyptian women: A cross cultural study. *International Quarterly of Community Health Education, 4* (1), 77-83.

Engs, R.C. (1983). The health concerns of students and the implication for alcohol education programming. *Journal of Alcohol and Drug Education, 29,* (1), 36-39.

Engs, R.C. (1970). *The health concern questionnaire.* University of Oregon, Eugene.

Goodrow, B. (1977, May/June). Does time change the health concerns of college students? *Health Education, 34-35.*

Norusis, M.J. (1987). The SPSS guide to data analysis for SPSSX. SPSS: Chicago, Illinois.

Table 1

Forced 2 Factor Solution Using (Varimax Rotation)
Eigenvalue Minimum of 2 for Testing
Construct Validity (N=388)

Factor	Eigenvalue	% of Variance	Correlation Coefficient Between Factor 1 & 2
1	16.6	33.3	.58
2	3.3	6.7	
3	1.9	3.8	
4	1.8	3.5	
5	1.5	3.0	
6	1.4	2.9	
7	1.3	2.5	
8	1.2	2.3	
9	1.1	2.1	

Table 2

Mean Score and Standard Deviation of All 50
Items Ranked by Descending Score

Item		Mean	Standard Deviation
1.	AIDS	3.5	1.2
2.	Cancer	3.3	1.1
3.	What I'll be like in 10 or 15 years	3.3	1.2
4.	Birth Control	3.3	1.2
5.	Auto Accidents	3.3	.9
6.	Use of Contraceptives	3.1	1.2
7.	Death	3.1	1.3
8.	Sexually Transmitted Disease other than AIDS	3.0	1.3
9.	Overweight	2.9	1.4
10.	Nuclear Warfare	2.9	1.1
11.	Heart Disease	2.8	1.2
12.	Childbirth	2.8	1.3
13.	Smoking and Disease	2.7	1.3
14.	Pregnancy	2.7	1.4
15.	Sex Behavior	2.6	1.5
16.	Halitosis (bad breath)	2.5	1.3
17.	Acne	2.4	1.1
18.	Alcohol Dependence	2.4	1.1
19.	Poor Teeth and Decay	2.4	1.2
20.	Nervousness	2.3	1.0
21.	Moodiness	2.3	1.0
22.	Eye Disorders and Blindness	2.3	1.2
23.	Biological and Chemical Warfare	2.3	1.2
24.	Air Pollution	2.3	1.0
25.	Being Burned	2.3	1.1
26.	Suicide	2.3	1.0

Item	Mean	Standard Deviation
27. Water Pollution	2.3	1.3
28. Drowning	2.2	1.2
29. Starvation and Malnutrition	2.2	1.2
30. Airplane Accidents	2.2	1.1
31. "Colds"	2.2	1.2
32. Sterility	2.2	1.0
33. Drug Abuse	2.2	1.0
34. Emphysema or Respiratory Disease	2.1	1.2
35. Firearm Accidents	2.1	1.3
36. Combat	2.1	1.2
37. Headache	2.0	1.0
38. Homosexuality	2.0	1.3
39. Kidney Disease	2.0	1.0
40. Mental Illness	2.0	1.1
41. Mononucleosis ("mono")	2.0	1.0
42. Radiation	2.0	1.0
43. Liver Disease	2.0	1.0
44. Nausea	1.8	1.0
45. Population Explosion	1.8	1.0
46. Accidents due to Electric Current	1.7	1.0
47. Tuberculosis ("TB")	1.6	0.9
48. Riots	1.6	0.9
49. Poisoning by Snakes	1.5	0.9
50. Masturbation	1.3	0.7

INDEX

A

Adaptation to aging, 191
Adolescent condom use, 71
Adolescent drug use, 5
Adolescent health education priorities, 155-174
Adolescent HIV-AIDS programs, 1-68
Adolescent pregnancy, 112
Adolescent's HIV-AIDS knowledge, 6-8
Age and preventive health behaviors, 203-213
AIDS prevention, 69-100
American Red Cross HIV-AIDS Program, 12
American School Health Association, 155
Argentine hemorrhagic fever, 215-230
Attitudes and behavior, 176
Attitudes toward premarital intercourse, 114
Attitudes toward sex, 116-118
Attitudes towards sexuality in life, 114

B

Barriers to smoking cessation, 239
Behavior attitudes, 72
Behavioral intent, 233-234
Bloom's Taxonomy of Educational Objectives, 144

C

Caring for skin, 160
Centers for Disease Control, 103
Child abuse, 166
Cigarette smoking and morbidity, 232
Clarity of personal sexual values, 114
Clinic records, 292
Cognitive tasks in health education, 141
Communication about HIV-AIDS, 28-29
Condom use against HIV, 71
Condom use by high school students, 69-100
Contraceptive practices of adolescents, 4-5